W9-DAS-307

WITHDRAWN

Is the World Prepared for a Deadly Influenza Pandemic?

Scott Barbour

INCONTROVERSY

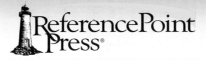

ReferencePoint
Press®

San Diego, CA

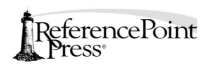

© 2011 ReferencePoint Press, Inc.

For more information, contact:
ReferencePoint Press, Inc.
PO Box 27779
San Diego, CA 92198
www. ReferencePointPress.com

Picture credits:
Cover: iStockphoto.com
AP Images: 9, 24, 28, 31, 37, 41, 46, 64, 69, 74, 79
Landov: 22
Photoshot: 49, 56
Science Photo Library: 7, 16

LIBRARY OF CONGRESS CATALOGING-IN-PUBLICATION DATA

Barbour, Scott, 1963-
  Is the world prepared for a deadly influenza pandemic? / by Scott Barbour.
    p. cm. — (In controversy)
  Includes bibliographical references and index.
  ISBN-13: 978-1-60152-127-9 (hardback)
  ISBN-10: 1-60152-127-8 (hardback)
  1. Influenza—Epidemiology—Popular works. I. Title.
  RA644.I6B37 2010
  614.5'18—dc22
                                                       2010005

Contents

Foreword

I n 2008, as the U.S. economy and economies worldwide were falling into the worst recession since the Great Depression, most Americans had difficulty comprehending the complexity, magnitude, and scope of what was happening. As is often the case with a complex, controversial issue such as this historic global economic recession, looking at the problem as a whole can be overwhelming and often does not lead to understanding. One way to better comprehend such a large issue or event is to break it into smaller parts. The intricacies of global economic recession may be difficult to understand, but one can gain insight by instead beginning with an individual contributing factor such as the real estate market. When examined through a narrower lens, complex issues become clearer and easier to evaluate.

This is the idea behind ReferencePoint Press's *In Controversy* series. The series examines the complex, controversial issues of the day by breaking them into smaller pieces. Rather than looking at the stem cell research debate as a whole, a title would examine an important aspect of the debate such as *Is Stem Cell Research Necessary?* or *Is Embryonic Stem Cell Research Ethical?* By studying the central issues of the debate individually, researchers gain a more solid and focused understanding of the topic as a whole.

Each book in the series provides a clear, insightful discussion of the issues, integrating facts and a variety of contrasting opinions for a solid, balanced perspective. Personal accounts and direct quotes from academic and professional experts, advocacy groups, politicians, and others enhance the narrative. Sidebars add depth to the discussion by expanding on important ideas and events. For quick reference, a list of key facts concludes every chapter. Source notes, an annotated organizations list, bibliography, and index provide student researchers with additional tools for papers and class discussion.

The *In Controversy* series also challenges students to think critically about issues, to improve their problem-solving skills, and to sharpen their ability to form educated opinions. As President Barack Obama stated in a March 2009 speech, success in the twenty-first century will not be measurable merely by students' ability to "fill in a bubble on a test but whether they possess 21st century skills like problem-solving and critical thinking and entrepreneurship and creativity." Those who possess these skills will have a strong foundation for whatever lies ahead.

No one can know for certain what sort of world awaits today's students. What we can assume, however, is that those who are inquisitive about a wide range of issues; open-minded to divergent views; aware of bias and opinion; and able to reason, reflect, and reconsider will be best prepared for the future. As the international development organization Oxfam notes, "Today's young people will grow up to be the citizens of the future: but what that future holds for them is uncertain. We can be quite confident, however, that they will be faced with decisions about a wide range of issues on which people have differing, contradictory views. If they are to develop as global citizens all young people should have the opportunity to engage with these controversial issues."

In Controversy helps today's students better prepare for tomorrow. An understanding of the complex issues that drive our world and the ability to think critically about them are essential components of contributing, competing, and succeeding in the twenty-first century.

Preparing for the Inevitable

On June 11, 2009, the World Health Organization (WHO), the division of the United Nations responsible for monitoring global health and disease, announced that the world was at the start of an influenza pandemic. The disease was called H1N1, after its scientific designation, but was often referred to as swine flu due to the belief that it originated on a pig farm. H1N1 first appeared in Mexico in late April, and by the time of WHO's announcement, there were 30,000 confirmed cases in 24 countries. At a press conference announcing her decision to declare the outbreak a pandemic, Margaret Chan, WHO's director general, stated, "Further spread is considered inevitable."[1]

A Worldwide Problem

By definition, a pandemic is a disease outbreak that spreads to all parts of the world. It is different from an epidemic, which is a disease outbreak that is confined to a smaller area, such as a community, a country, or even one continent. To be declared a pandemic, the disease does not need to kill large numbers of people; it only needs to be a disease that spreads worldwide.

An influenza pandemic can be relatively mild or extremely severe, depending on the genetic makeup of the virus strain. The virus must be easily transmitted from person to person in order to spread worldwide, but it need not be particularly deadly. Experts typically discuss the severity of influenza pandemics by comparing them to one another, as there have only been a few influenza pandemics in recent history from which to gather statistics. The deadliest influenza pandemic by far was the 1918–1920 Spanish flu pandemic, which killed between 40 million and 100 million people worldwide. By comparison, the 2009 outbreak was mild, killing 12,220 people by the end of 2009. In fact, the H1N1 pandemic proved to be far less deadly than even the seasonal (non-pandemic) influenza, which kills between 250,000 and 500,000 people every year.

Although the H1N1 pandemic was relatively benign, public health experts analyzed the global reaction to the outbreak to determine whether the United States and the rest of the world would be prepared in the event of a truly deadly influenza pandemic. In the United States various organizations and government agencies conducted reviews of the U.S. government's response to the H1N1 outbreak and reached varying conclusions.

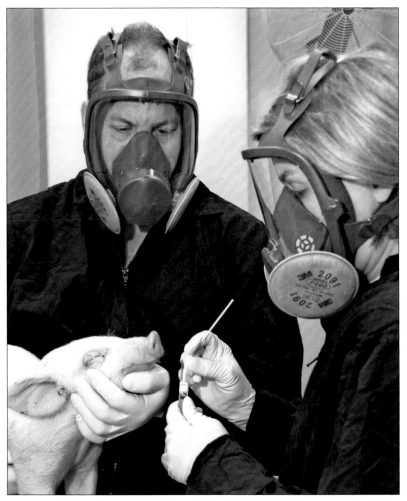

Medical researchers take a nasal swab from a piglet to test for the H1N1 influenza virus. Authorities believe H1N1, also called swine flu, originated on a pig farm. The first confirmed cases of the virus in humans were found in Mexico.

The consensus was that the country's readiness for an influenza pandemic had improved in recent years but that more improvements were needed—for example, in the areas of vaccine development and coordination between government and nongovernment agencies. The conclusions of the President's Council of Advisors on Science and Technology (PCAST), a group of scientists and engineers who advise the U.S. president, were representative. PCAST found that "the response was probably the best effort ever mounted against a pandemic" but cautioned that "some aspects of the decision-making and preparation process . . . could be improved."[2]

More Pandemics Are Inevitable

While America—along with the rest of the world—escaped disaster in 2009, the H1N1 outbreak underscored the fact that the threat of an influenza pandemic is constant. As stated by Michael T. Osterholm, a professor of public health at the University of Minnesota, "Like earthquakes, hurricanes, and tsunamis, influenza pandemics are recurring natural disasters."[3] The question is not *if* another influenza pandemic will occur, but *when.* In addition to being inevitable, influenza pandemics are unpredictable—both in their timing and their severity. The deadliness of a pandemic depends primarily on the genetic makeup of the virus—a factor over which humanity has absolutely no control.

"Like earthquakes, hurricanes, and tsunamis, influenza pandemics are recurring natural disasters."[3]

— Michael T. Osterholm, professor of public health at the University of Minnesota.

Public health experts contend that high-level planning is the key to minimizing the extent of illness and death that a truly deadly pandemic would cause. At the international level, WHO conducts constant surveillance of influenza virus mutations and disease outbreaks. In addition, WHO advises governments on how best to plan for an influenza pandemic. Its *Checklist for Influenza Pandemic Preparedness Planning* includes a comprehensive list of steps divided into sections such as: preparing for an emergency; surveillance; case investigation and treatment; preventing the spread of the disease in the community; maintaining essential services.

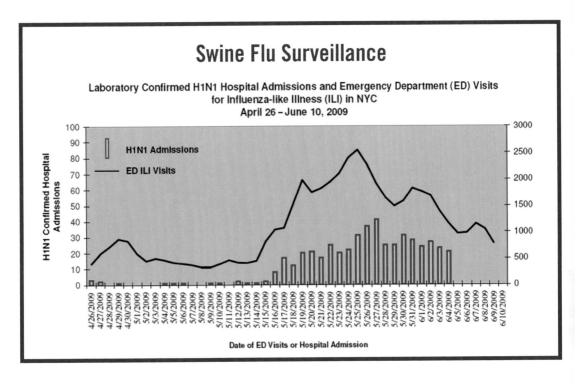

Swine Flu Surveillance

Laboratory Confirmed H1N1 Hospital Admissions and Emergency Department (ED) Visits for Influenza-like Illness (ILI) in NYC
April 26 – June 10, 2009

The Challenges of Planning Ahead

In the United States the Department of Health and Human Services has devised a *Pandemic Influenza Plan* that addresses the steps outlined by WHO. The plan lays out in great detail actions to be taken by specific government agencies prior to and during an influenza pandemic. For example, before a pandemic, the government is to partner with other nations to conduct ongoing surveillance and early detection of pandemic viruses. In addition, it must ensure that the nation's hospitals and other treatment providers are able to increase their capacity to receive and treat a sudden upsurge in the number of patients.

Once a pandemic virus has been identified, the government must determine whether to impose travel restrictions, school closures, or other community-based measures to limit the spread of the disease. Officials must inform the public of the crisis in a manner that will encourage compliance with official recommendations without inciting panic. In addition, the government must decide whether to release antiviral drugs from the Strategic National Stockpile in order to control the spread of the disease as well as to

During the 2009 swine flu pandemic, health departments around the country charted the number of emergency room visits for influenza-like illnesses. This type of information helps public health officials track rates and severity of influenza and also adjust hospital staffing where needed. The graph shows the number of people with flu symptoms who visited hospital emergency rooms in New York City between April 26 and June 10, 2009.

treat symptoms and perhaps save lives. At the same time, officials must collaborate with private industry in the development and production of a vaccine for the new virus.

As this description suggests, responding to an influenza pandemic is a major undertaking. Most experts agree that the world is better equipped than ever to respond to a truly deadly outbreak, but more could be done. Thus officials will continue to improve their plans and develop their medical and public health capabilities in anticipation of the next pandemic. As stated by Osterholm: "The world will experience another pandemic, and it will get through it, as it has all previous ones. The challenge is to figure out now how to minimize the number of deaths and the economic and psychological devastation it will cause."[4]

Facts

- According to the U.S. Department of Health and Human Services, the next influenza pandemic will likely originate overseas, not in the United States.

- Once infected with influenza, children "shed" the virus in larger amounts than adults, thus making them more contagious.

What Is the History of Influenza Pandemics?

Between 1918 and 1920 a severe and fatal disease swept the globe. The pandemic, described by the President's Council of Advisors on Science and Technology as "the worst natural calamity of the twentieth century,"[5] took an enormous toll on individuals and families. Debbie Crane relates the story her grandmother, Edna Breedlove Clampitt, told her about surviving the scourge as it ravaged North Carolina:

> By mid-December, the whole family was terribly ill. They ached. Their throats hurt. They coughed and coughed. My great-grandmother, Ida Mae Breedlove, gave birth even as she lay sick. My grandmother described one terrible night when the whole family sounded as if they were all drowning. In the morning, Ida and 2-year-old Woodrow were dead. The newborn, named Paul, died days later.[6]

The illness that struck the Breedlove family—influenza, or flu—is an infectious respiratory illness caused by a virus. There are three types of the influenza virus: A, B, and C. All three types can infect humans; however, only type A can cause a pandemic. Type B causes severe illness and death in humans but only mild epidemics (not pandemics). Type C causes only mild illness in people.

Of the three types of influenza virus, only type A is further classified into different subtypes. Scientifically, subtypes of the type A influenza virus are denoted by a series of letters and numbers that refer to their genetic makeup, such as H1N1 or H5N1. They are also commonly named after the animal to which they are most closely linked. For example, H1N1 is often called swine flu, whereas H5N1 is referred to as bird, or avian, flu.

Drift and Shift

The influenza virus incubates primarily in birds before spreading to other animals such as pigs and to people. The risk from influenza lies in its ability to mutate—that is, its ability to change its genetic makeup and develop into different strains. A strain is a finer variation than a type or subtype. Thus, while the type B virus has no subtypes, it does evolve into different strains (as do the subtypes of the type A virus). This is the process by which the viruses stay one step ahead of the human body's immune system.

Influenza strains develop by means of 2 processes known as antigenic drift and antigenic shift. Antigenic drift is the process by which type A and B influenza viruses undergo gradual mutations as they copy themselves during the reproductive process. The word *antigenic* refers to the body's immune response; thus the phrase *antigenic drift* refers to genetic changes that create new virus strains to which humans are not immune. Because humans lack an antigenic response, the new strain spreads easily and may cause an epidemic, a disease outbreak that affects a large number of people within a community. Antigenic drift is responsible for the seasonal flu, a nonpandemic form of the disease that affects 5 to 20 percent of the global population and leads to 200,000 hospitalizations and approximately 36,000 deaths in the United States each year.

In addition to antigenic drift, the type A influenza virus (but not types B or C) is capable of antigenic shift, also known as reassortment. Type A viruses contain eight genes. When two different type A viruses infect the same cell, they can trade genes, creating a new virus subtype. Typically this trade involves a strain of avian flu or swine flu exchanging genes with a strain of human flu. Because the new virus is so drastically different than either of the previous viruses, the human immune system has little or no defense against it. As stated by WHO, "If this new 'hybrid' virus contains the right mix of genes, causing severe disease and allowing easy and sustainable human-to-human transmission, it will ignite a pandemic."[7] In fact, new type A influenza subtypes created via antigenic shift are responsible for all of the known influenza pandemics in history. There is no way to know when such a shift will occur; thus, influenza pandemics are completely unpredictable.

Infection and Mortality Rates

Influenza pandemics typically occur in waves of varying severity. The number of people infected—known as the infection rate or morbidity rate—is higher in a pandemic than in an annual seasonal flu outbreak. While seasonal flu infects 5 to 20 percent of the population, pandemic flu infects about 30 percent of the population. The rate at which the virus spreads—the transmission rate—is also higher with pandemic influenza. The transmission rate for the seasonal flu is between 1.1 and 1.8, which means that an infected person will spread the virus to between an average of 1.1 and 1.8 people. In a pandemic, the transmission rate is between 1.5 and 5.5. Because older people have usually been exposed to various influenza subtypes in their childhoods, they typically have more immunity to new viruses and are less likely to be infected than are younger people.

The rate of fatalities—known as the mortality rate—for pandemic flu is also typically higher than for seasonal flu. The case mortality rate for the seasonal flu is 1 per 1,000, meaning that 0.1 percent of people who are infected die. By contrast, during the Spanish flu pandemic, 2.5 percent of those who contracted the disease died. The mortality rate also varies from pandemic to pandemic due to variation in the virus strains' transmission rate and virulence—that is, its ability to overcome the body's natural defenses.

Discovery of the Virus

No one is sure when the first influenza pandemic occurred. Historians have identified several large outbreaks suspected of being in-

"If [a] new 'hybrid' [influenza] virus contains the right mix of genes, causing severe disease and allowing easy and sustainable human-to-human transmission, it will ignite a pandemic."[7]

— The World Health Organization, the branch of the United Nations responsible for monitoring and responding to global health crises.

Can Masks Stop the Spread of Influenza?

Influenza is transmitted from person to person primarily by means of large, virus-laden droplets. When a person with influenza coughs or sneezes, these droplets travel through the air, potentially coming in contact with the upper respiratory tract of anyone nearby. Contact typically occurs through the nose or mouth; once that happens, infection is likely to occur. During the 2009 H1N1 pandemic, people in many countries donned masks in an attempt to prevent infection. These masks are also routinely used by medical personnel who come in close contact with ill patients. According to the Centers for Disease Control and Prevention (CDC), no studies have proven that masks are effective in preventing influenza infection. Nevertheless, the CDC recommends that medical personnel use a mask while within 3 feet (0.91m) of a person with a respiratory disorder such as influenza. During the H1N1 pandemic, the CDC said there was no need for most people to wear masks in public, at work, or at home. However, the agency suggested that people at high risk for severe complications consider wearing a mask when in a crowded setting or when caring for a person with influenza-like illness.

fluenza between the sixteenth an[...] effects & [...]ing to Mark Honigsbaum, an autho[...] casualties on [...]s in the history of diseases, it was n[...] mass scale [...]mic of 1889 to 1890, which killed a[...]hat scientists became alarmed abou[...]sed this pandemic has not been id[...]nfident that it was in fact a strain[...]tes: "Whereas before 1889 most do[...]rely mild and harmless, after 1889 medical professionals had little choice but to take it seriously."[8]

Prior to the twentieth century, experts believed influenza was spread by various means. In the seventeenth century, epidemics were believed to be caused by volcanic eruptions and the passage of meteors. In fact, the word *influenza* is believed to come from the Italian phrase *influenza coeli*, which means "influence of the heavens." In the eighteenth century, influenza was believed to be caused by cold. The Italian phrase *influenza di freddo*, which means "influence of the cold," was used to describe the illness. In the nineteenth century, scientists made many advances, including the discovery of bacteria and their role in illnesses such as tuberculosis and cholera. Thus it was assumed that influenza was spread in the same way. It was not until 1933 that scientists discovered the cause of influenza when they isolated the virus that had led to the Spanish flu pandemic of 1918 to 1920.

The Spanish Flu Pandemic

Of the 4 confirmed influenza pandemics, the Spanish flu pandemic of 1918 to 1920 was the first and by far the most severe. It infected 25 to 30 percent of the world's population and killed between 40 million and 100 million people (more than died in World Wars I and II combined), including 500,000 to 750,000 in the United States, 250,000 in Britain, and 50,000 in Canada. The name of the Spanish flu is a fluke of history. Because the illness appeared during World War I, most nations hesitated to report plague deaths in order to conceal the fact that their armies were weakened and thus vulnerable to attack. Spain was not a party to the conflict and therefore had no qualms about publicizing the illness sweeping through its population. Thus the name *Spanish flu* stuck, even though the origins of the disease remain unknown.

The illness struck young people especially hard. Most older people had encountered a similar strain of flu earlier in their lives, so their bodies had developed partial immunity to the virus. Young people had no such immune defense. Therefore, when confronted with the new infectious agent, the bodies of many younger people mounted an extreme immune response which often killed them

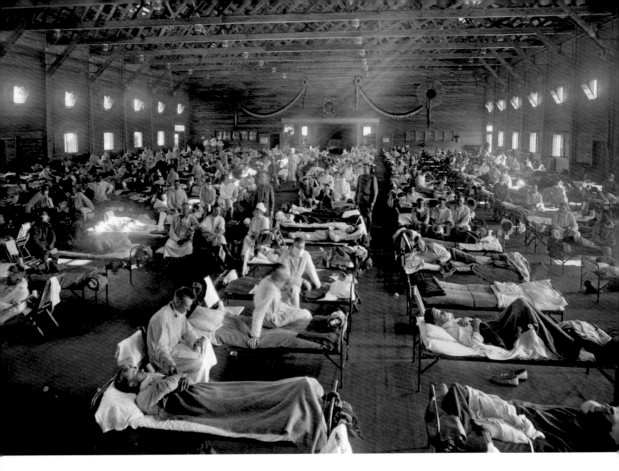

Hundreds of patients receive care at an emergency hospital ward set up at a U.S. Army camp in Kansas during the 1918 Spanish flu pandemic. Forty million to 100 million people worldwide died from Spanish flu during the pandemic.

by filling their lungs with fluids, essentially drowning them. Honigsbaum describes a typical case of Spanish flu:

> "Spanish" influenza struck suddenly and without warning: one moment a person was up and about, the next they would be lying incapacitated coughing up greenish-yellow sputum. In some cases, a frothy, blood-stained fluid gushed from their nose and mouth. As pneumonia set in their temperature would soar to 40 or 41° C [Celsius; 104 to 106° Fahrenheit] and they would slip into a delirium. The final stage came when their lungs filled with fluid prompting their heart to leech oxygen from the blood vessels supplying the head and feet. . . . Typically, a blue or dark-purple stain would spread across the lips and cheekbones. Then the victim would turn a mahogany colour and die.[9]

Responding to the Crisis

The first wave of the disease to sweep the globe, in the spring of 1918, was relatively mild. However, the second wave, in the summer of 1918, was deadly. The virus had a transmission rate of about 3.0, meaning that each person who contracted the virus spread it to 3 other people. This high transmission rate allowed the illness to spread easily and to kill large numbers of people, leading to civil unrest and even rioting. The virus spread especially fast among American troops living in close quarters and being deployed across the Atlantic in ships. About 43,000 soldiers died of the disease in 3 months. So heavy were the fatalities that the transport vessels became known as "death ships." Laurie Garrett, an author and journalist who specializes in the history of diseases, explains how the depletion of military personnel impeded the government's ability to respond to the outbreak: "By late September 1918, so overwhelmed was the War Department by influenza that the military could not assist in controlling civic disorder at home, including riots caused by epidemic hysteria. Worse, so many doctors, scientists, and lab technicians had been drafted into military service that civilian operations were hamstrung."[10]

Although experts mistook the cause of the disease—believing it to be a bacterium rather than a virus—civic leaders took measures to control its spread. In the United States some cities quarantined sick patients; closed schools, theaters, and churches; and discouraged other social gatherings. These measures are often referred to as nonpharmaceutical (nondrug) interventions (NPIs), social containment measures, or social distancing. Recent studies have compared transmission and mortality rates in cities with and without NPIs during the pandemic. They have found that these efforts were effective while they were in place. Cities that imposed NPIs early in the pandemic had fewer deaths and lower transmission rates than cities that imposed no NPIs or imposed NPIs later in the pandemic. However, because governments were overwhelmed by the magnitude of the crisis, they were unable to sustain these controls, and the virus quickly regained ground when the NPIs were removed.

"'Spanish' influenza struck suddenly and without warning: one moment a person was up and about, the next they would be lying incapacitated coughing up greenish-yellow sputum."[9]

— Mark Honigsbaum, journalist and author of *Living with Enza: The Forgotten Story of Britain and the Great Flu Pandemic of 1918.*

The devastation wrought by the Spanish flu was epic in proportion. While it struck down millions in the developed nations, the disease ravaged less developed countries even harder. For example, 5 percent of the population of Ghana and 20 percent of the population of Western Samoa were killed by the disease. Entire Inuit villages were reportedly wiped out. These statistics, along with the details of the virus's capacity to inflict suffering, fuel alarm about the possibility of another deadly pandemic.

Two More Twentieth-Century Pandemics

Following the Spanish flu pandemic, there were 2 additional pandemics in the twentieth century. The first was the Asian flu pan-

Why Was the Spanish Flu So Deadly?

Scientists have long puzzled over why the Spanish flu pandemic of 1918 to 1920 was so deadly, killing as many as 100 million people worldwide. One group of researchers infected mice with a reconstructed strain of the 1918 virus and found that they had an extreme immune response that left them vulnerable to secondary illness. In essence, the body was trying so hard to kill the virus that it ended up damaging itself and leaving itself vulnerable to secondary infections such as pneumonia.

Another group of researchers, using ferrets as subjects, isolated a set of three genes that they believe combined to give the virus its deadly power. Most flu viruses reproduce in the upper respiratory tract—the mouth, nose, and throat. However, the researchers discovered that the Spanish flu virus contained three genes that, working together with another key gene, allowed the virus to replicate in the lungs as well as in the upper respiratory tract. This ability to reproduce in the lungs, experts believe, left victims more vulnerable to pneumonia and therefore increased the lethality of the virus.

demic of 1957 to 1958. By the time the Asian flu arrived, the world was much better prepared for a pandemic. The viral cause of influenza had been discovered, vaccines for seasonal flu had been used for years, and antibiotics had been developed to treat secondary pneumonia, which is often the cause of flu fatalities. In addition, WHO, which was established in the late 1940s, had created an influenza surveillance system in 1947. As a result, WHO quickly detected the virus and alerted governments to begin producing vaccines and preparing for large numbers of flu patients. However, while a vaccine was available by the late summer and fall of 1957, the number of doses was limited by lack of production capacity.

In the absence of adequate doses of vaccine, some countries instituted social containment measures such as school closures and travel restrictions. However, according to WHO, these efforts merely delayed, rather than prevented, the spread of the illness due to the highly contagious nature of the virus. Though it was a less virulent strain than the Spanish flu, the Asian flu killed about 2 million people globally, including 70,000 in the United States.

The third and final influenza pandemic of the twentieth century was the Hong Kong flu pandemic of 1968 to 1970. As its name suggests, this virus originated in Hong Kong. The virus spread much more slowly than the Asian flu and proved much less severe. The Hong Kong flu killed about 1 million people globally, including 34,000 Americans. Researchers believe that the Hong Kong flu virus was similar to a virus already in circulation, which may have resulted in partial immunity among the population and therefore a lower death rate.

The Swine Flu Scare of 1976

A few years after the Hong Kong flu, in 1976, experts became alarmed by the appearance of a new strain of the virus that was responsible for the Spanish flu pandemic. In January of that year, several army recruits at Fort Dix in New Jersey fell ill, and 1 died. Fearing a repeat of the Spanish flu pandemic, in March 1976 U.S. president Gerald Ford called for a program to inoculate all Americans against the virus.

The effort got underway, and about 25 percent of the population (45 million people) received the vaccine that fall. However, the program was suspended after about 500 people who had received the vaccine developed a disorder known as Guillain-Barré syndrome (GBS), a neuromuscular condition that causes paralysis. Of those struck by GBS, 25 died. The role of the vaccine in causing the GBS cases remains unclear, and the number of people affected was small (about 1 in 100,000, or 0.001 percent of those who received the vaccine) when compared with the number who could be saved by a vaccine in the event of an influenza pandemic. However, because no pandemic ever came—raising the possibility that people were harmed unnecessarily—the vaccine effort was viewed as a disaster.

The 1976 swine flu scare may have had lasting consequences in terms of undermining the public's trust in the government to deal with a major disease outbreak. It had an especially negative effect on the government's ability to persuade people that influenza vaccines are safe. As Michael Specter writes in the *New Yorker*, "The episode helped establish a widespread fear of vaccines that . . . persists to this day. More than that, it created a false sense, shared by millions, that vaccines were at least as threatening as the diseases they prevent."[11]

The H5N1 Outbreak

As the 1976 scare illustrates, prior to the 1990s governments mostly reacted to pandemics rather than prepared for them. This situation changed around the turn of the twenty-first century, when a virulent strain of H5N1 began to kill people in Asia, Europe, and Africa. Although the virus was extremely deadly—killing 60 percent of those infected—it did not develop the ability to be transmitted from person to person. Because the transmission of the virus was limited to bird-to-human contact, mainly infecting people in Southeast Asia who lived in close proximity to fowl, H5N1 did not cause a pandemic. However, the virus has continued to spread to various parts of the world, carried by wild migratory birds and passed on to domesticated

"The [1976 influenza vaccination] episode helped establish a widespread fear of vaccines that . . . persists to this day. More than that, it created a false sense, shared by millions, that vaccines were at least as threatening as the diseases they prevent."[11]

— Michael Specter, staff writer at the *New Yorker* magazine and author of *Denialism: How Irrational Thinking Hinders Scientific Progress, Harms the Planet, and Threatens Our Lives.*

fowl such as ducks and chickens. Moreover, it continues to infect and kill humans. According to WHO, as of December 30, 2009, 467 cases of H5N1 had been reported in 15 nations; 282 (60 percent) of these cases had resulted in death. The countries with the largest number of H5N1 cases were Indonesia, Vietnam, and China, but by 2009 the disease had spread throughout the Middle East and Asia.

Because of its extremely high fatality rate, public health officials were concerned that the H5N1 virus could prove catastrophic if it developed the ability to be transmitted from human to human and spread worldwide. The U.S. government took several steps to prepare for the possibility of a deadly influenza pandemic. In November 2005 President George W. Bush issued the National Strategy for Pandemic Influenza, which outlined measures for the United States to prepare for a pandemic, including the stockpiling of medical supplies and antiviral drugs; expanding the capacity to produce more vaccine doses more quickly; and improving surveillance, communication, and containment efforts.

In 2006 Bush released the Implementation Plan for the National Strategy for Pandemic Influenza, a blueprint with more than 300 recommendations for influenza preparedness and response. He asked Congress for $7.1 billion to fund the effort. While Congress did not approve the full amount, it did pass the Pandemic Influenza Act of 2006, which authorized $3.3 billion for influenza preparedness. As a result, the nation's ability to produce antiviral drugs and vaccines was greatly increased, and the medical and public health agencies had clearer guidelines on how to respond to a pandemic. Other countries—including Australia, Canada, Japan, and the United Kingdom—developed similar plans.

The Swine Flu Pandemic of 2009

The world's preparations for a pandemic were put to the test beginning in March and April 2009, when a new strain of the H1N1 virus emerged in Veracruz, Mexico. By the end of April, there were 1,918 suspected cases and 97 laboratory-confirmed cases of illness caused by the new strain; 84 patients had died.

Early in the outbreak, officials were alarmed by the number of deaths among young people in Mexico. However, the virus turned out to be less deadly than initially feared. Nevertheless, the disease posed a significant threat of serious illness and death to certain groups of people, especially young people, pregnant women, and those with underlying medical conditions. A study of 642 patients early in the outbreak found that 60 percent were age 18 or younger; only 5 percent were older than 50. Pregnant women accounted for 13 percent of deaths among H1N1 patients early in the outbreak. People with heart disease, lung disease, and diabetes, along with those suffering from obesity, HIV, and other illnesses, also proved more susceptible to illness and death.

Early in the outbreak, WHO called for the production of a vaccine for the new virus strain, but the first doses were not

A sign urges visitors at an Alabama hospital to use hand sanitizer during the H1N1 pandemic. Such dispensers were installed at locations around the United States. Authorities in Mexico also urged use of hand sanitizers during the pandemic.

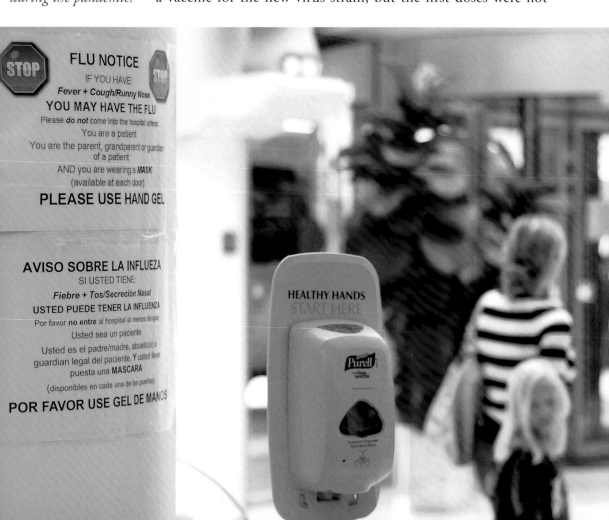

available until October. In the meantime, governments responded to the emergence of the new virus strain in different ways. In the first weeks Mexico closed all schools in its capital city and advised incoming airline passengers to seek medical treatment if they developed symptoms. Mexican officials also launched a massive media campaign, distributed masks and alcohol-based hand sanitizer to the public, and discouraged public gatherings such as church services, theater events, and soccer games. On April 27 all schools in Mexico were ordered closed.

Other nations also took dramatic steps in response to the outbreak. In Egypt officials slaughtered thousands of pigs due to the erroneous belief that they were the cause of the disease. In the United States about 600 schools in 19 states were temporarily closed in response to H1N1 infection among students. In Tokyo citizens donned surgical masks before venturing out in public in hopes of preventing the spread of flu germs. In May WHO announced that attempts to contain the virus by means of travel restrictions were not feasible and recommended no such restrictions be imposed. The United States heeded WHO's advice. However, other countries, most notably China, suspended flights and quarantined foreigners suspected of being infected with the virus or having come in contact with infected persons.

On June 11, 2009, WHO declared the outbreak a pandemic due to its presence in at least 2 regions of the world. However, in the fall of 2009 health officials began reassessing the response as it became clear that the pandemic was not as severe as first thought. Revised guidelines were issued, and school closures were kept to a minimum. According to WHO, as of December 27, 2009, H1N1 had been reported in 208 countries or territories and had resulted in more than 12,220 deaths.

> "[Health authorities] simply called attention to the potential threat of the [2009 H1N1] pandemic and began preparing for it. This is what we pay them for."[12]
>
> — Arthur Allen, author of *Vaccine: The Controversial Story of Medicine's Greatest Lifesaver.*

Assessing the Response

Reaction to the U.S. government's handling of the 2009 pandemic has been mixed. Some contend that the government (and WHO) overreacted to the emergence of the H1N1 virus, sowing unnecessary fear and provoking excessively costly responses. For

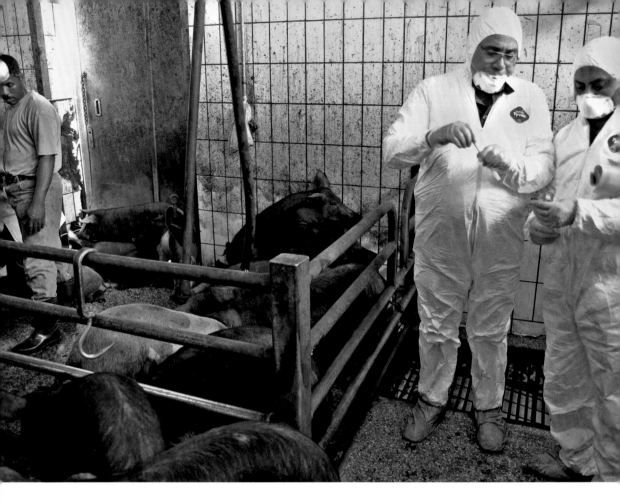

An Egyptian medical team examines pigs about to be slaughtered in April 2009. Government officials ordered the slaughter of 300,000 pigs as a precaution against swine flu. The action was later condemned as unnecessary.

example, in October President Barack Obama declared the pandemic a national emergency despite a relatively low death rate. Others insist that due to the unpredictability of the virus, health officials responded appropriately. As stated by Arthur Allen, the author of *Vaccine: The Controversial Story of Medicine's Greatest Lifesaver*, health authorities "simply called attention to the potential threat of the pandemic and began preparing for it. This is what we pay them for."[12] Had the outbreak been more serious, the nation would have been better equipped to respond. Moreover, due to the government's response to the bird flu threat years before, the government was better prepared to produce vaccines, distribute antiviral drugs, and coordinate communications. Most agree that in the end, evaluations of the H1N1 pandemic—and the official response to it—will provide useful information for those who must prepare for the next deadly influenza pandemic.

Facts

- According to the World Health Organization, 99 percent of deaths during the Spanish flu pandemic occurred in people under age 65.

- A study conducted by researchers at both Harvard and Stanford universities found that the Spanish flu pandemic was number 4 on the list of economic disasters since 1870, behind World War I, World War II, and the Great Depression.

- Throughout history most influenza pandemics have started in areas where large numbers of people live in close proximity to fowl and pigs.

- The Hong Kong flu pandemic of 1968 to 1970 had a mortality rate of 0.01 percent, while the Spanish flu of 1918 to 1920 had a mortality rate of 2.5 percent.

- On average, there are three influenza pandemics per century, occurring 10 to 50 years apart.

CHAPTER TWO

Can Predictions Help the World Prepare for Future Pandemics?

Influenza pandemics are inherently unpredictable. As stated by WHO, influenza viruses are "sloppy, capricious, and promiscuous."[13] There is no telling when a new strain of type A influenza will emerge with the ability to spread from human to human and cause a pandemic. Some experts have pointed out that even weather-related events such as tornados and hurricanes are more predictable than influenza pandemics.

In addition to being unpredictable in their timing, influenza pandemics are unpredictable in their severity. There is no way to know ahead of time whether the next pandemic will be relatively mild, like the 1968 pandemic, or severe, like the 1918 pandemic—or worse. As WHO states, "The actual consequence of the next pandemic will be greatly influenced by the properties of the virus, which cannot be known in advance."[14]

The Importance of Assumptions and Predictions

Although the timing, severity, and impact of the next influenza pandemic cannot be known in advance, experts believe that, based on past pandemics, assumptions and predictions can be made to help the world plan and prepare for future pandemics. Researchers often use past influenza pandemics to generate scenarios regarding the number of people who would fall ill and die in pandemics of varying severity. They also study the potential effects of pandemics on the health-care system, the infrastructure (water, electric power, waste disposal, and so on), the economy, and national security. These scenarios and predictions are then used to guide officials in drawing up plans for their response to the medical, social, and economic consequences of the world's next influenza pandemic.

For example, estimates about the numbers of people who would become sick and die help the federal government lay the groundwork for the production of vaccines, the distribution of antiviral drugs, and the timing of social containment measures such as school closures and travel restrictions. Such estimates can also help the government craft communications that effectively inform the public of the true nature of the threat in a way that does not incite panic.

On a more local level, estimates of casualties allow health-care agencies to plan for the number of hospital beds, surgical masks, respirators, and other crucial supplies they will need and to make contingency plans to ramp up their staffs of doctors, nurses, and volunteers. Local public health officials can use assumptions and estimates about pandemics to prepare their plans for distributing vaccines, educating the public, and guiding school districts and businesses regarding the advisability of closing or remaining open. Thus assumptions, predictions, and scenarios, however inexact they may be, are crucial tools in the effort to prepare for a potentially deadly influenza pandemic.

Assumptions About the Next Pandemic

The U.S. Department of Health and Human Services (HHS) has made numerous assumptions about the next influenza pandemic. According to the HHS, everyone will be susceptible to the new virus strain. The attack rate (the proportion of people who will become infected) will be about 30 percent, and about 50 percent of those infected will seek medical care, causing a surge in the need for medical supplies and personnel. Within any community, an outbreak will last from 6 to 8 weeks. There will most likely be at least 2 waves of disease outbreak, and once the pandemic has ended, the new virus strain will continue to circulate as part of the seasonal virus.

Other assumptions carry less certainty due to the variations seen in past pandemics. For example, the number of people who will require hospitalization or who will die will depend on the virulence of the new strain of influenza. In addition, the groups of people who will be most at risk of illness and death is dependent on the virus strain and the degree of immunity to it among the public. Influenza typically targets the very young, the very old, and those who are already sick. However, the 1918 virus struck young, healthy people the hardest; the 2009 H1N1 virus also attacked young people harder than the elderly. The rate of spread of the new virus is also impossible to predict, with estimates that each infected person will pass the virus on to 2 or 3 people.

A teenager who has a rare genetic disorder is treated for H1N1 symptoms in the intensive care unit of a Chinese hospital in August 2009. Most flu viruses have the strongest effect on the very young, the very old, and those who are already sick.

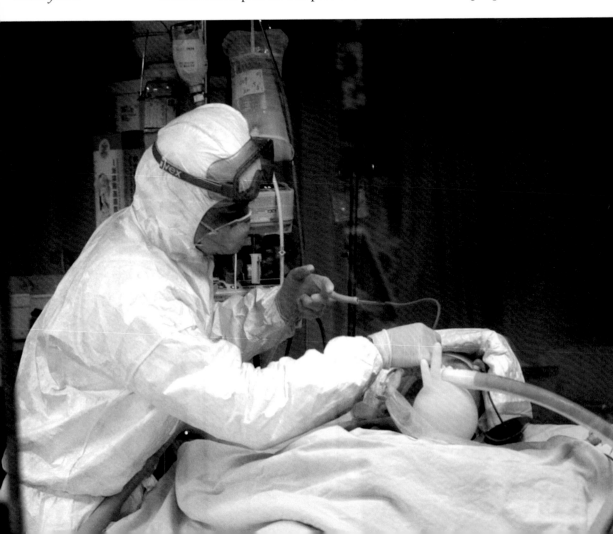

Scenarios of Morbidity and Mortality

In addition to assumptions, public health experts also rely on scenarios, or hypothetical descriptions of events, to help them estimate the consequences of pandemics and prepare an adequate response. Estimates of the number of people who would become sick and die (morbidity and mortality) as a result of a pandemic vary. The HHS estimates that a severe outbreak similar to the 1918–1920 virus could result in 10 million hospitalizations and 1.9 million deaths in the United States; a moderate outbreak similar to the 1968–1970 virus could result in more than 800,000 hospitalizations and 200,000 deaths. However, the HHS notes that these numbers do not factor in the possible impact of interventions such as antiviral and antibacterial drugs that are now available; thus the numbers could be considerably lower.

To get a picture of the global impact of an influenza pandemic, economists Warwick J. McKibbin and Alexandra A. Sidorenko created a computer model to study 4 scenarios: a mild pandemic similar to the Hong Kong flu of 1968 to 1970, a moderate pandemic similar to the Asian flu of 1957 to 1958, a severe pandemic similar to the Spanish flu of 1918 to 1920, and an ultra pandemic even more serious than the Spanish flu. The researchers concluded that a mild pandemic would cause 1.4 million deaths (20,000 in the United States); a moderate pandemic would cause 14 million deaths (200,000 in the United States); a severe pandemic would cause 71 million deaths (1 million in the United States); and an ultra pandemic would cause 142 million deaths (2 million in the United States).

Effects on the Health-Care System

The quick spread of a new influenza virus strain would place a heavy burden on the health-care system, including hospitals and emergency rooms. Additional pressure would be placed on public health agencies responsible for informing the public, coordinating the distribution of vaccines and antiviral drugs, and overseeing social containment measures such as school closures or quarantines. Experts predict that in a severe pandemic, the capacity of hospital emergency rooms (their "surge capacity") would be tested. Many hospitals would not have enough beds to handle the patient load. According to the Congressional Budget Office, an independent agency that provides economic data to Congress, "A severe pandemic in an urban area would increase the overall demand for beds and staff three times beyond the current capacity and the demand for intensive care beds seven times beyond the current capacity."[15] Besides beds and staff, hospitals would also need additional equipment, including respirators, ventilators, surgical masks, gloves, and gowns.

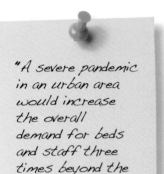

Hospital staffing would also be strained during a deadly influenza pandemic. In the United States the health-care system is currently experiencing a nursing shortage of 100,000 in the absence of a major pandemic. Faced with a severe outbreak, demand for staff would go up while nurse absenteeism would also rise due to illness, the need to stay home and care for children, and fear of contracting the disease. An April 2009 survey of health-care union representatives conducted by the AFL-CIO, a labor union organization, found that many health-care workers believed their workplaces were not prepared to handle an influenza pandemic. As a result of this lack of preparedness, 43 percent of those surveyed believed that "most or some members will stay home"[16] from work in order to protect themselves and their families from infection. Such absenteeism could have a major impact on the ability of the system to respond to a major pandemic.

Effects on Infrastructure and Social Stability

Predictions vary on the effects that a deadly pandemic could have on society. With large numbers of people sick and dying, businesses, governments, and schools could be significantly impacted. Many people would be absent from work and school due to illness, death, or caring for sick family members. This high absenteeism could drastically affect the functioning of businesses and government, as well as the provision of basic services. Energy, water, waste disposal, transportation, and other essential services could be drastically disrupted. As stated by the Homeland Security Council, an agency within the White House that advises the president on homeland security issues, "While a pandemic will

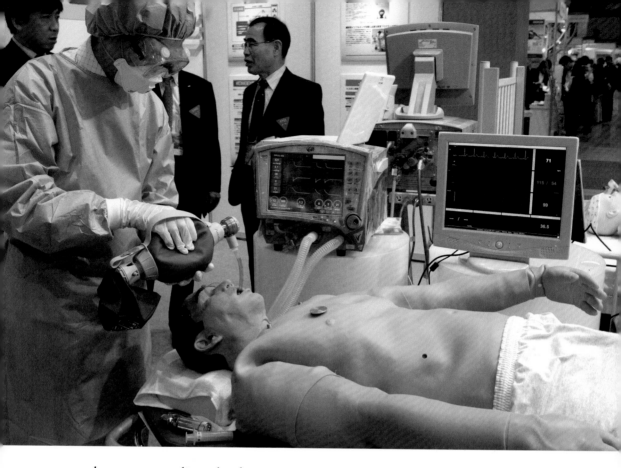

not damage power lines, banks or computer networks, it will ultimately threaten all critical infrastructure by removing essential personnel from the workplace for weeks or months."[17]

As the infrastructure and economy break down, a severe pandemic could lead to social unrest. Illness in their families, combined with a shortage of goods and services, could cause people to panic. Geary W. Sikich, an author who specializes in business crisis management, describes a possible scenario of societal breakdown:

> People are less patient, are more stressed, and have a greater tendency to act out their frustrations than ever before. In a pandemic, the stress level will be even greater because of the uncertainty of whether or not one will become infected. . . . There will be panic as people rush to stockpile essential items, such as food and water. More panic will emerge as people find that medicines that are now more regulated are unavailable.[18]

A technician demonstrates the use of a human patient simulator designed to help medical workers diagnose and treat influenza patients. Like a person infected with the H1N1 virus might do, the robotic patient sweats, cries, moans, and convulses.

WHO Advocates Scenarios for Influenza Preparedness

In July 2009 the World Health Organization (WHO) issued guidelines for influenza pandemic preparedness in the nonhealth sector. WHO stresses that an influenza pandemic could adversely impact every sector of society, including business, transportation, and the provision of basic services such as food and water. As one of five principles of readiness for global, national, and local influenza pandemic preparedness, WHO stresses the importance of scenarios:

> The impact of an influenza pandemic on specific communities will vary from mild to severe, depending on vulnerability and capacity to respond. Therefore, it is appropriate to develop and plan for different scenarios that may arise, using clearly defined planning assumptions. Plans should consider what actions would be implemented in the event of these different scenarios. It is important to be clear what actions will be taken should the worst case scenario materialize. It is prudent to plan for the worst, while hoping for the best.

World Health Organization, "Whole-of-Society Pandemic Readiness," July 2009. www.who.int.

In an extreme scenario, there is even the possibility that riots could break out, necessitating the use of social control measures such as curfews and National Guard troops to impose order.

The Effects on the Economy

In addition to its impact on infrastructure and social stability, a pandemic would have a negative effect on the economy due to the removal of so many people from the labor force. A pandemic would also harm the economy by causing a reduction in the consumption of goods and services, an increase in business operating costs, and a disruption of international trade. As McKibbin and Sidorenko state, an influenza pandemic would cause "a decline in the size of the labor force due to a rise in mortality and disabling illness, an increase in the cost of doing business, especially in the service sector . . ., a shift in consumer preferences away from services that require exposure to other people . . ., [and] a re-evaluation of investment risk."[19] The degree of the impact on the country's economy depends on the virulence of the virus and the degree of the country's exposure to the disease.

McKibbin and Sidorenko used a computer model that included 20 countries or regions (the United States, Japan, Europe, and others) and 6 sectors of the economy (energy, mining, agriculture, durable-goods manufacturing, nondurable goods manufacturing, and services). The equations used in the model factored in the trade and financial market linkages between and within economies and the shocks to the system from a pandemic. They examined the effect of a pandemic on each nation's gross domestic product (GDP), the value of all the products and services the nation produces in one year. The researchers found that, not surprisingly, the more severe the pandemic, the more severe the impact on the economy. A mild pandemic would reduce the GDP of the United States by 0.6 percent; a severe pandemic would reduce it by 3.0 percent. Other countries would be more severely impacted. For example, a severe pandemic would shrink the GDP of the Philippines by 19.3 percent. In the ultra scenario, the global GDP is reduced by 12.6 percent, or $4.4 trillion. The authors conclude:

> Even a "small" pandemic would generate hundreds of billions in losses—and a disproportionate amount of those losses would be borne by the developing countries, which could least afford the blow. At least one conclusion, then, is crystal clear: it would pay to invest considerable resources now to prevent a flu pandemic and to prepare for the consequences of massive economic jolts if the pandemic does come.[20]

"Even a 'small' pandemic would generate hundreds of billions in losses—and a disproportionate amount of those losses would be borne by the developing countries, which could least afford the blow."[20]

— Warwick J. McKibbin, professor at Australian National University College of Business and Economics, and Alexandra A. Sidorenko, adjunct research fellow at Australian National University.

Other researchers have found similar results. For example, in 2006 the Congressional Budget Office found that a mild pandemic would reduce the GDP of the United States by about 1 percent, while a severe pandemic would reduce the GDP by 4.25 percent. However, the Congressional Budget Office stresses that the impact would be temporary: "In each case, economic activity would probably snap back once the pandemic ended, as consumers increased spending and businesses increased production to meet pent-up demand."[21] Other experts foresee more severe long-term consequences to the economy, including a global depression. As stated by Sikich: "We are likely to see a depression or an extremely prolonged period of economic stagnation. . . . The socioeconomic picture does not look to be good right away in the post-pandemic timeframe."[22]

Effects on National Security and Global Stability

Besides its economic impact, an influenza pandemic could have a major effect on U.S. national security. Members of the military would be among those to become ill and die in a pandemic, thus weakening the armed forces. In addition, as Sikich writes, even a mild pandemic "could cause degradation to our national security because of the shifting of our focus from dealing with threats such as terrorism to dealing with the socioeconomic disruption created by media-driven panic."[23] Some commentators even suggest that an influenza virus could be intentionally introduced into society in an act of terrorism or that terrorists could strike during a pandemic, when the nation would be especially vulnerable. As explained by the majority staff of the U.S. House of Representatives Committee on Homeland Security:

An enemy could take advantage of the next influenza pandemic to increase the force of an attack by combining the pandemic with intentionally-introduced diseases and epidemics. An enemy could also take other actions to hasten the spread of strains of influenza that are thought to be harbingers of the pandemic. . . . It is also likely that terrorists would recognize that hospitals and other critical infrastructures would become even more appealing targets during a pandemic.[24]

The risk to U.S. national security could be made worse by worldwide instability. Many countries around the world, especially developing nations, lack stable governments and efficient infrastructures (electricity, water, transportation, and so on) to begin with. In addition, many of them depend on aid from nongovernmental institutions such as the World Bank, the International Monetary Fund, and the United Nations. In the event of a

Could 1918 Happen Again?

Much of the discussion about the threat of a deadly influenza pandemic centers on the possibility of an outbreak as severe as the Spanish flu of 1918 to 1920. Some experts contend that another outbreak of this magnitude is almost certain. They point out that a virus with the virulence of the 1918 bug could quickly spread to all parts of the world by means of air travel. Others reject this possibility. They point out that in 1918, knowledge of viruses was nonexistent. Today the viral cause of influenza is known, and vaccines and antiviral drugs can be used to combat the disease. Moreover, improvements in health care, such as the use of ventilators and antibacterial drugs to treat pneumonia, can also help prevent deaths. Finally, disease surveillance systems and global communications networks would quickly alert the entire world to the outbreak and keep even the most remote areas of the planet informed about the virus and how to control it. Referring to the Spanish flu pandemic, Philip Alcabes, a professor of urban public health at the City University of New York, states, "We'll never see another flu outbreak of that sort."

Philip Alcabes, "5 Myths About Pandemic Panic," *Washington Post*, March 15, 2009, p. B-3.

pandemic, some or all of this support could be withdrawn, leading to the degradation of infrastructure and a decreased quality of life, which in turn could provoke rioting, the rise of paramilitary or revolutionary forces, armed conflict, and weakened or failed governments.

With the American government and military weakened and the world in chaos, the United States could face threats from new sources. As Sikich explains: "A pandemic could lead to a degradation of U.S. power and the rise of regional power centers. . . . Competing power centers may attempt to challenge the United States in the belief that the United States, weakened by a pandemic, could be opposed effectively. . . . This could lead to extreme global geopolitical instability."[25] In addition, a pandemic could provoke armed conflict between nations currently or historically at odds, such as India and Pakistan or China and Taiwan.

An Inexact Science: A Scenario That Was Wrong

Scenarios of the effects of an influenza pandemic are hypothetical. They are educated guesses based on past events and current knowledge. The scenarios are not intended to predict the future; they are meant to serve as tools to help society, the health-care system, and the government to prepare. An example that proves the fallibility of scenarios took place during the H1N1 outbreak of 2009.

On August 7, 2009, the President's Council of Advisors on Science and Technology (PCAST) issued a scenario for the second wave of the H1N1 virus expected to sweep the United States in the fall. PCAST was adamant that its forecast was a scenario of what could potentially happen, rather than a prediction of what would definitely happen. In PCAST's scenario, the virus in the fall would be as virulent as in the previous spring, but its transmission rate would be higher. It would infect 30 percent to 50 percent of the population (90 million to 150 million Americans); about 1 million to 2 million people would require hospitalization; and 30,000 to 90,000 people would die of the virus. In fact, this scenario proved wrong. While the virus did return in the fall, it was quite mild and resulted in relatively few hospitalizations

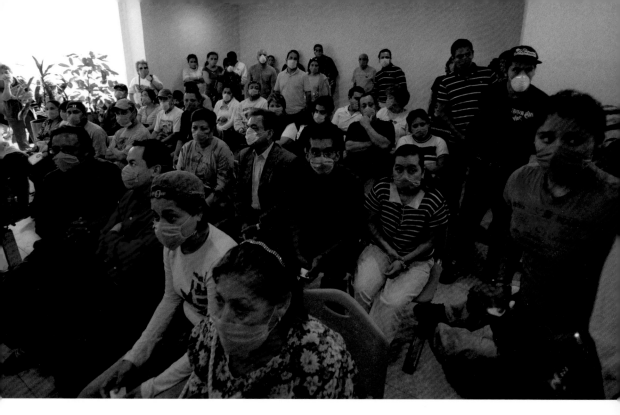

and deaths. Although exact statistics are not available, the Centers for Disease Control and Prevention estimates that between April and October 2009, there were 98,000 hospitalizations and 3,900 deaths due to H1N1 in the United States, figures much lower than PCAST's estimates.

The waiting room of a Mexico City hospital fills with people waiting to be seen at the height of the 2009 H1N1 scare. Part of planning for a deadly flu pandemic includes determining whether hospital emergency rooms can handle a higher-than-normal patient load.

Preparing for Pandemic or Inciting Panic?

Some commentators cite PCAST's off-base scenario as evidence of how public health experts and the media exaggerate the threat of pandemics and incite widespread panic. Writing in October 2009, Michael Fumento, an author who specializes in science and health issues, said: "What we're seeing is pandemic panic. . . . Scared people are indeed swamping emergency rooms, and schools are closing. But it's not flu-driven; it's fear-driven. The media write articles about panicky people, thereby creating more panicky people."[26]

Others were less critical of PCAST and other officials who expressed concern about the possibility of a deadly fall wave of H1N1. The *Christian Science Monitor*, a daily national newspaper, stressed PCAST's insistence that their estimate was a plausible scenario on which to base its plans, not a prediction, a subtle distinction that the media failed to communicate. In defense of PCAST, the *Christian Science Monitor* said, "The federal government seems to be striking the right balance—steering the public away from alarm, while trying to plan and prepare."[27] Others contend that due to the uncertainty surrounding the risk of pandemic influenza, it may be acceptable to err on the side of caution—or even panic. Anne Applebaum, a columnist for the *Washington Post*, states, "Where infectious diseases are concerned, panic is good. Panic is what we want. Without panic, nothing happens."[28] She cites the example of malaria, a disease that continues to kill a million people a year—due, she says, to a lack of hysterical media coverage.

Weighing the Costs of Preparedness

Most experts agree that more influenza pandemics are inevitable. What cannot be known in advance are two of the most important aspects of a pandemic: its timing and its severity. As Laurie Garrett puts it, "Evolution does not function on a knowable timetable, and influenza is one of the most mutation-prone pathogens in nature's storehouse."[29] Despite these unknowns, public health experts can rely on assumptions and scenarios in an attempt to plan and prepare for the next crisis.

Unfortunately, planning and preparing for a severe pandemic is expensive. During a time of recession, when many governments are forced to cut back, pandemic preparedness may take a backseat to more immediate concerns. As WHO says, governments are forced to ask, "What priority should be given to preparedness for an inevitably recurring event of unpredictable timing and an outcome that is also unpredictable but could be catastrophic?"[30] Faced with this dilemma, some governments may choose to forgo influenza pandemic planning. This failure to heed the lessons of the past and invest in preparedness could result in major loss of life along with substantial social and economic disruption. As stated by Michael T. Osterholm, "In a world filled with competing international priorities, preparing for something that may not happen in the next year may seem hard to justify in terms of both financial resources and time, but that is no excuse for inaction."[31]

Facts

- **Historically, border closures and travel restrictions have slowed the spread of pandemic influenza but have failed to stop it.**

- **A study published by the Australian Treasury found that an influenza pandemic with a mortality rate one-third that of the Spanish flu of 1918 to 1920 would reduce Australia's gross domestic product by nearly 6 percent.**

- **A study published by the Canadian Department of Finance found that a pandemic with mortality rates similar to the 1918–1920 Spanish flu pandemic would reduce the gross domestic products of industrialized nations such as Canada and the United States by 0.3 to 1.1 percent.**

- **A 2003 outbreak of severe acute respiratory syndrome (SARS), a respiratory illness that, like influenza, is caused by a virus, killed 775 people and cost the world an estimated $40 billion.**

- **An October 2009 poll by Rasmussen Reports found that 66 percent of Americans believe the media made the threat of swine flu sound worse than it actually was.**

Is the Global Pandemic Response System Adequate?

O ne of the most important tools in the fight against a deadly influenza pandemic is information. The timely gathering and effective dissemination of data is crucial in order to mobilize resources, coordinate the official response, and inform members of the public of the threat and the steps they must take to protect themselves and their loved ones.

In the event of a flu pandemic, information must travel many directions at once. Individual nations are expected to inform the rest of the world of flu activity within their borders. This data must be compiled and sent back to public health agencies at the national, state, and local levels. Government offices, schools, and businesses must be informed of potential closures or other protective measures. Physicians and other health-care providers must be kept up to date on symptoms, diagnosis, and treatment protocols. Finally, individual citizens must be informed of the threat and the appropriate response by means of media broadcasts, public service announcements, and other methods. All of this information must be delivered in a way that is consistent and measured in order to prevent panic.

The Importance of WHO

The most important source of information related to influenza is the World Health Organization (WHO), a division of the United

Nations that is responsible for monitoring threats to global health and coordinating the international response. Emphasizing the importance of WHO in the event of a flu pandemic, *Washington Post* columnist Anne Applebaum states:

> The WHO may well be the only international organization that we cannot live without. When infectious diseases are spread rapidly across borders, WHO is expected to coordinate the scientific response of national public health officials, from France to Malaysia, as well as the global information campaign needed to explain it. No national government can do the same.[32]

Thousands line up for H1N1 flu vaccination in Idaho in October 2009. A sign warns those who already have flu symptoms to see their doctors rather than seek the vaccine.

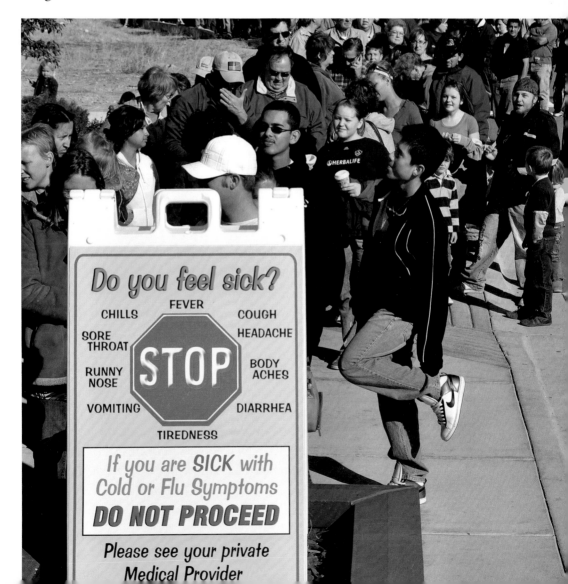

Do you feel sick?

CHILLS · FEVER · COUGH
SORE THROAT · HEADACHE
STOP
RUNNY NOSE · BODY ACHES
VOMITING · DIARRHEA
TIREDNESS

If you are **SICK** with Cold or Flu Symptoms
DO NOT PROCEED
Please see your private Medical Provider

One of WHO's functions is to conduct surveillance, sometimes called "biosurveillance," in order to detect and trace viruses as they change. To this end, all nations are expected to report influenza-related illnesses and deaths to WHO. In addition, WHO oversees a network of 130 institutions in 101 countries that test patients with influenza-like illness and submit samples to WHO's laboratories for analysis. Each year, more than 175,000 patient samples are collected, and about 2,000 viruses are submitted to WHO for testing. This analysis allows WHO to determine whether new viruses are emerging as well as whether existing vaccines are effective.

This massive undertaking relies on individual nations to voluntarily report information. However, many nations lack sophisticated virus surveillance systems—especially poor, rural regions, where new flu viruses are most likely to spring up. This deficiency in detection and reporting capabilities undermines WHO's ability to stay on top of viruses and react swiftly to new threats. As stated by Lawrence Gostin, a professor of global health law at Georgetown University, "Many poor countries lack adequate surveillance, early warning systems and modern laboratories; they also have negligible public health infrastructures."[33] He points out that the developed nations, such as the United States, have done little to help poor nations develop their capacity to detect and respond to the flu, leaving the whole world vulnerable. To address these vulnerabilities, WHO is seeking to expand the coverage of its network and to make better use of electronic communications technologies in order to obtain real-time information about the mutation of viruses and the spread of diseases.

WHO's Phase System

In addition to the surveillance of influenza, WHO is responsible for alerting nations of threats posed by new flu strains that are or may become pandemic. In order to communicate the level of pandemic hazard efficiently to all countries at once, WHO relies on a phase system consisting of 6 levels, with phase 6 being a pandemic. Under WHO's phase system, phases 1 and 2 are the interpandemic period, or the period between pandemics. Phases 3 through

"The WHO may well be the only international organization that we cannot live without."[32]

— Anne Applebaum, columnist for the *Washington Post* newspaper.

5 are the pandemic alert period. Phase 3 is declared when a new virus strain has emerged; phase 4 when small clusters of humans have become infected; and phase 5 when large clusters of humans have become infected but the spread remains localized. Phase 6 is the pandemic period. In order to reach phase 6, the virus must be easily passed from human to human and must be present in at least 2 of 6 regions of the planet: Africa, the Americas, the Eastern Mediterranean, Europe, Southeast Asia, and the Western Pacific.

WHO's phase system was criticized during the 2009 H1N1 pandemic. WHO declared the H1N1 outbreak a phase 6 pandemic on June 11, 2009, stating that the disease had sustained human-to-human transmission and had spread to at least 2 WHO-designated regions of the globe. However, at that time, only 144 people had died after contracting the H1N1 virus. In subsequent weeks and months, the swine flu proved to have a

Triage in an Influenza Pandemic

During a severe influenza pandemic, hospitals would likely be swamped with a surge of patients experiencing varying degrees of illness—from the "worried well" (those who are not sick but think they are) to the severely ill and dying. Hospitals may lack the personnel or other resources—such as ventilators and antiviral drugs—needed to treat such an influx of patients adequately. Faced with this dilemma, they may be forced to perform triage, a technique in which patients are divided into categories and given a higher or lower priority status. Those with no chance of survival would likely be given minimal treatment. Similarly, those likely to survive without treatment would also receive little care. Highest priority would be given to patients with serious illness who have a good chance of survival with treatment. While denying people treatment may seem harsh, the goal of triage is to make the most of available resources and save as many lives as possible.

high transmission rate—that is, it spread easily from person to person—but a low mortality rate. In fact, it turned out to be less fatal than the seasonal flu, which has led to suggestions that WHO's definition of *pandemic* might need to be changed. As stated by the Trust for America's Health, a nonprofit organization that advocates policies to protect public health, "The WHO pandemic alert phase system was not well matched with the realities of the H1N1 outbreak, since most of the planning . . . focused on the geographic patterns, but not the severity of the disease."[34]

Should Pandemic Be Redefined?

Critics cited two problems with declaring H1N1 a pandemic. First, because WHO declared it a pandemic, the public might not take WHO's warnings seriously when deadlier diseases emerge in the future. Second, WHO's pandemic declaration signaled the nations of the world to activate their pandemic response plans. These plans varied from nation to nation, but generally included costly measures such as the stockpiling of medical supplies, the distribution of vaccines, and the mobilization of public health resources that inconvenienced the public and had a negative impact on businesses and national economies.

Some critics contend that WHO's definition of *pandemic* should be revised to account for the severity of the flu strain. Only a highly virulent virus that sickens and kills large numbers of people should qualify as a pandemic, they suggest. However, most epidemiologists insist that WHO's definition is accurate and should not be changed. The word *pandemic* refers to a disease that has a global reach regardless of its lethality, they point out. Vincent Racaniello, a virus researcher at the Columbia University College of Physicians and Surgeons, states: "WHO redefining pandemic is absurd. Pandemic is an epidemiological definition that has nothing to do with virulence."[35] In fact, *Webster's Dictionary* defines a pandemic as a disease occurring over a wide area and affecting a large proportion of people; it says nothing about mortality rates.

Despite disagreements over its phase system, WHO remains the world's best defense against a deadly flu pandemic. However,

WHO has limited power and must rely on voluntary cooperation of nations rather than the force of international law. According to Gostin, "The frightening truth is that the WHO has no real power. It lacks an effective mechanism for monitoring and enforcing national reporting. Its recommendations to countries are expressly 'non-binding.' Countries do not even have to share virus samples with it."[36] Gostin and others insist that WHO should be given more authority in order to compel international cooperation in the event that the world is faced with a truly deadly influenza pandemic.

International Cooperation Crucial

The importance of international cooperation in the face of pandemics is illustrated by 2 examples. The first involves the 2002–2003 outbreak of severe acute respiratory syndrome (SARS). SARS is similar to influenza in that it is a potentially fatal viral respiratory disease. Between November 2002 and July 2003, an outbreak of SARS originated in China and spread to about 37 countries, infecting over 8,000 people and killing more than 700. Although it never reached pandemic status, the SARS outbreak is often cited as an example of what can go wrong when a nation withholds information from WHO. Although the first victim of SARS died in November 2002, China did not report the death to WHO until February 2003. In the meantime, the Chinese took actions to control and conceal the outbreak. Unfortunately, this delay in reporting the disease also postponed WHO's response to it, placing additional lives in jeopardy.

A more recent example that illustrates the importance of international cooperation involves the Southeast Asian nation of Indonesia. In 2007 Indonesia's health minister, Siti Fadilah Supari, announced that her country would stop providing WHO with samples from people who have become ill or died from avian influenza, an extremely deadly strain of H5N1. Currently, bird flu mostly infects birds; however, it does spread to humans who come into close contact with infected birds, usually in the slaughtering process. Many public health experts believe that avian influenza

"The frightening truth is that the WHO has no real power. It lacks an effective mechanism for monitoring and enforcing national [influenza] reporting."[36]

— Lawrence Gostin, professor of global health law at the Georgetown University Law Center.

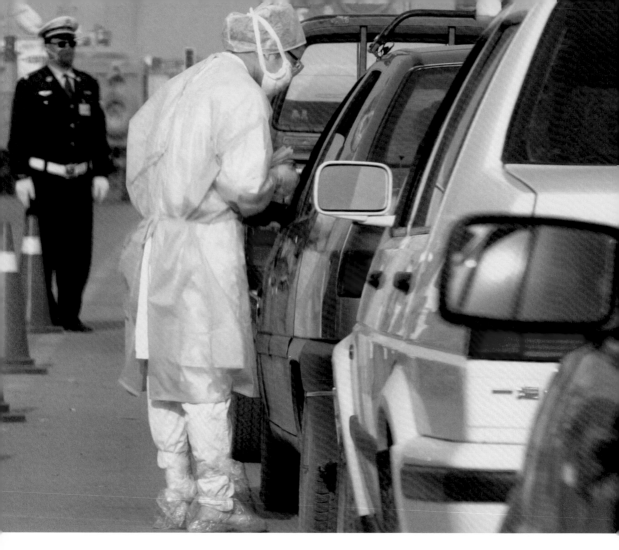

Even as they concealed information about the deadly SARS outbreak, Chinese authorities tried to control its spread. One measure involved medical workers interviewing drivers and checking their temperature at a checkpoint (pictured) before allowing them to proceed.

could develop the ability to spread from human to human and result in a disastrous pandemic. Because a large proportion (32 percent) of bird flu cases occurs in Indonesia, most experts consider the Indonesian government's cooperation with WHO critical in order to prevent a potential catastrophe.

Viral Sovereignty

The Indonesian government defends its policy on the grounds of "viral sovereignty"—that is, viruses that occur in Indonesia belong to the Indonesian people. The Indonesians have accused WHO of abetting rich nations in a plot to use virus samples to develop biological weapons as well as to sicken people in poor nations in order to profit from the sales of vaccines. Since Indonesia's announcement that it will withhold samples, other nations have endorsed the concept of viral sovereignty. In 2009 Indonesia's new health minister, Endang Rahayu Sedyaningsih, vowed to continue withholding virus samples unless poor countries were guaranteed equal access to vaccines.

The vast majority of public health experts reject Indonesia's claims, as well as the concept of viral sovereignty. They insist that the Indonesians are placing humanity at risk by withholding essential information. As stated by Richard Holbrooke, president of the Global Business Coalition on HIV/AIDS, Tuberculosis and Malaria, and Laurie Garrett, senior fellow for global health at the Council on Foreign Relations, "The failure to share potentially pandemic viral strains with world health agencies is morally reprehensible. Allowing Indonesia and other countries to turn this issue into another rich-poor, Islamic-Western dispute would be tragic—and could lead to a devastating health crisis."[37]

U.S. Surveillance and Response

While WHO leads the international response to influenza pandemics, each nation has its own public health agencies that coordinate activities within its borders. In the United States the agency responsible for flu surveillance is the Centers for Disease Control and Prevention (CDC). The CDC gathers and analyzes information on influenza in the United States and produces weekly reports. In total, the CDC surveillance system consists of about 150 laboratories (many in collaboration with WHO), 3,000 outpatient care sites, over 100 statistics offices, and epidemiologists from health departments in every U.S. state and territory. The CDC gathers 5 categories of data: viral surveillance, outpatient illness surveillance, mortality surveillance, hospital surveillance, and summaries of the geographic spread of influenza as reported weekly by state health departments. These sources of data allow the CDC to study when and where influenza activity is occurring, track influenza-related illness, determine which influenza viruses are circulating, detect changes in

Bird Flu in Indonesia

Avian influenza (H5N1, or "bird flu") has hit Indonesia harder than any other country. As of December 2009 the nation had experienced 141 confirmed human cases, 115 (82 percent) of which resulted in death. Experts believe that due to poor reporting, the actual numbers may be much higher.

One reason for the severity of the epidemic in Indonesia may be the fact that many Indonesians own chickens and allow them to wander freely through their homes and yards. According to a former agriculture official, the country has 1.4 billion chickens, 80 percent of which live in 395 million residences. These chickens are vital to the livelihood of many Indonesians. As explained by Seth Mydans, a journalist for the *New York Times*, "Household chickens serve as a small bank account for poor Indonesians." The chickens can be used for food, but they can also be sold for about $2 a piece when the family needs cash. Because chickens play such a crucial role in the economy, efforts to combat the bird flu virus have proved unsuccessful. Consequently, the virus continues to spread among birds and occasionally to people—giving it more opportunities, experts fear, to mutate into a pandemic strain.

Seth Mydans, "Indonesian Chickens, and People, Hard Hit by Bird Flu," *New York Times*, February 1, 2008, p. A-3.

influenza viruses, and measure the number of influenza-related deaths in the United States.

As part of its effort to help communities respond to a pandemic virus, in 2007 the CDC introduced a Pandemic Severity Index (PSI). This tool is designed to address the issue that pandemics can vary in their severity of symptoms and numbers of deaths. Modeled on the hurricane warning system, the PSI has 5 levels. Level 1 is mild and is used for a pandemic about as severe as the seasonal flu. More specifically, a level 1 pandemic would have a case mortality of 0.1 percent or less (that is, 0.1 percent or fewer of those infected would die) and would cause a total of fewer than 90,000 deaths. Level 5 is severe and would be used for a pandemic as serious as the 1918 Spanish flu pandemic. A level 5 pandemic would have a case mortality rate of at least 2 percent and would cause a total of 1.8 million deaths. Based on this rating, the 2009 H1N1 pandemic qualified as a level 1 pandemic.

In addition to the CDC, the U.S. Department of Health and Human Services (HHS) plays a major role in pandemic flu preparedness and response. In 2005, following the bird flu scare, HHS created a national Pandemic Influenza Plan to guide the

Chickens are killed and cut up for distribution at a New York City live-bird market. Similar markets in Southeast Asia are likely places for the spread of avian influenza from birds to humans.

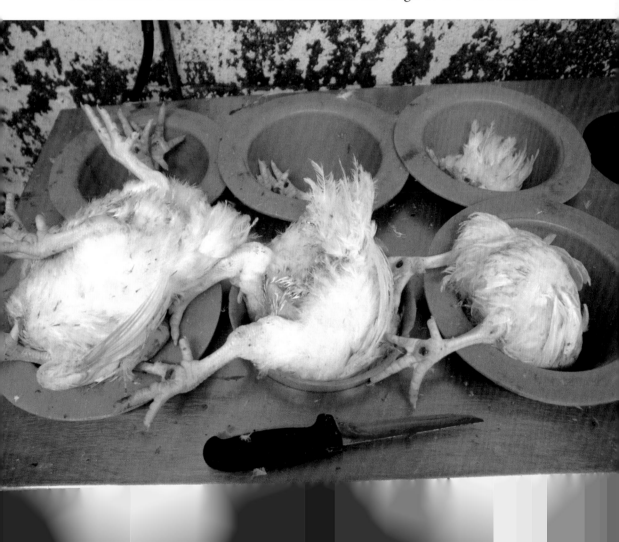

federal government's response to an emerging pandemic. The plan outlines key actions to be taken by the federal government in the face of a pandemic, including surveillance, protective public health measures, vaccine and antiviral drug production, health-care emergency response, and communications and public outreach. The plan also provides specific guidance to state, local, and tribal governments on how to respond to a pandemic. The HHS plan has 7 stages that correspond to WHO's 6 pandemic phases. Each action to be taken by the government is determined by the WHO phase of the pandemic. For example, during stages 2–3, which corresponds with WHO's phases 5–6 (pandemic alert and pandemic periods), the federal government may take steps to "potentially restrict arrivals to a limited number of U.S. ports of entry" and "evaluate travelers who are ill; isolate them and arrange for treatment, if necessary,"[38] according to the HHS.

U.S. Readiness

While the United States has comprehensive pandemic plans in place, it remains to be seen whether the nation is truly prepared for a deadly outbreak. One major challenge would be coordination of the various public health agencies. In addition to the CDC and HHS, the response to a deadly influenza pandemic would involve many other national agencies, including the U.S. Department of Transportation, the U.S. Food and Drug Administration, the U.S. Department of Agriculture, the U.S. Department of Homeland Security, and others. Defining which agency is responsible for which task can often be a challenge. These national agencies must in turn communicate and coordinate with state and local public health agencies, which in turn must coordinate with private health-care providers and the general public. Coordination of all these different organizations with varied tasks and responsibilities can be a challenge. For example, during the 2009 H1N1 pandemic, the Trust for America's Health found that "communication between the public health system and health providers was not well coordinated."[39]

In its evaluation of the U.S. government's response to the 2009 H1N1 pandemic, the President's Council of Advisors on Science and Technology found that "a well-defined process for decision making needs to be established well in advance, with clear assignment of responsibility and logical, agreed-upon guidelines for decision making."[40] The council concludes that in the United States, most decision making should fall to the U.S. Department of Health and Human Services.

In order to assess the federal government's readiness to respond to an influenza pandemic, in 2009 the General Accountability Office (GAO) surveyed the pandemic coordinators from 24 agencies regarding their operational plans. The GAO found that some agencies were more prepared than others to protect their workers and continue functioning in the event of a pandemic. For example, 19 of the agencies had plans to procure protective equipment such as masks and gloves for their employees, whereas only 11 had plans to make vaccines available to their workers. In order to address this inconsistency, the GAO recommended that the U.S. Department of Homeland Security be put in charge of monitoring and reporting to the president on the readiness of agencies to continue operations during a pandemic.

Surge Capacity

During a deadly pandemic, local health-care providers will be a key part of the response. Some public health experts fear that the health-care system is not prepared for such an event. Some worry that hospitals would be overwhelmed by sick and dying people and would be unable to care for them adequately due to a shortage of beds, supplies such as protective masks and ventilators, and personnel. This ability to handle a sudden onslaught of patients is commonly referred to as "surge capacity." In 2009 members of the U.S. House of Representatives Committee on Homeland Security stated, "Most hospitals in the country do not have the capacity to surge their operations to any great extent, so planners should not pretend that surge can occur easily."[41]

While the ability of U.S. hospitals to absorb a sudden surge cannot be completely known in advance, most experts agree that the nation's hospitals are better equipped than ever to withstand such a crisis. The U.S. Department of Health and Human Services

"Most hospitals in the country do not have the capacity to surge their operations to any great extent, so planners should not pretend that surge can occur easily."[41]

— U.S. House of Representatives Committee on Homeland Security, a committee of members of Congress that provides oversight of the U.S. Department of Homeland Security.

has provided more than $3 billion to state and local governments to develop their surge capacity. As a result, says Nicole Lurie, assistant secretary of preparedness and response for HHS, "Hospitals can now provide more beds; . . . track bed and resource availability . . .; protect their healthcare workers with proper equipment; decontaminate patients; . . . and coordinate regional training exercises."[42]

One factor that may impede the U.S. response to a pandemic is inadequate funding of public health agencies. While the U.S. government invested heavily in flu preparedness after the SARS outbreak of 2003 and the bird flu scare of 2005, investment has declined in recent years due to a global economic recession and the lack of an immediate threat. As Kim Krisberg, a writer for *Nation's Health* magazine, explains, "While the U.S. public health system has received millions in federal funds for emergency and pandemic flu preparedness since 2002, such funds have dwindled in the last few years and only worsened as states slashed their budgets to compensate for an ailing economy."[43] In the United States only 1 to 2 percent of health-care spending goes toward prevention and public health, which includes pandemic preparedness. Many experts contend that public health organizations such as the CDC and HHS must receive more funding.

A Global Issue

Protecting the world from a sneaky, mutating microbe is a huge challenge. The influenza virus does not recognize borders. Therefore, when it comes to pandemic prevention, the world truly is a global community. This fact is more evident today, in this era of easy air travel, than at any time in history. In the event of a deadly influenza outbreak, WHO will be called on to oversee humanity's response to the crisis, while national health organizations will be expected to cooperate with WHO, with one another, and with their own internal state and local health agencies. A massive, multidirectional flow of communication and coordination will be required among all parties—from national governments to state health agencies to hospitals to individual citizens—if humanity is to respond effectively to the threat, limit the number of deaths, and maintain global stability.

Facts

- After the World Health Organization raised the status of the H1N1 outbreak to phase 6, its highest level, in 2009, a poll by the Harvard School of Public Health found that 37 percent of Americans were more concerned about the disease, 6 percent were less concerned, and 57 percent reported no change in their level of concern.

- Despite improvements in surveillance and reporting of influenza viruses in recent years, it took three weeks for WHO to issue its first warning regarding the 2009 H1N1 virus after the first cases emerged.

- A 2009 survey published in the *American Journal of Public Health* found that 34 percent of adults were able to define *pandemic influenza* in a way consistent with the definition stated by WHO.

- In its communication response to an influenza outbreak, the Centers for Disease Control and Prevention is guided by several principles: acknowledging the situation early, maintaining transparency, identifying uncertainties and the unpredictable nature of influenza, and offering anticipatory guidance.

- According to the World Health Organization, the most important goal in communicating with the public during an influenza pandemic is gaining people's trust so they will follow instructions regarding disease prevention measures.

- Due to the communication efforts of the World Health Organization, UNICEF (the United Nations Children's Fund), and other international agencies, 70 percent of people in most countries with avian influenza outbreaks are aware of the disease; the rate is 90 percent in some countries, including Indonesia, Cambodia, and Thailand.

CHAPTER FOUR

Can Vaccines Prevent a Pandemic?

When the H1N1 virus was discovered in the spring of 2009, public health officials immediately ordered the production of massive doses of a vaccine against the new influenza strain. Unfortunately, the process involved in developing a vaccine requires months. That meant the public had to wait five months before the first vaccines were available—and even then, supplies were limited.

Despite the delay that developing a vaccine entails, most public health experts believe that a vaccine is humanity's best defense against a deadly influenza pandemic. Vaccination prevents a person from contracting and spreading the virus. Thus a vaccine is seen as the most effective way to control the spread of the disease and to limit the number of people who get sick and die.

Unlike pandemic flu vaccines, seasonal flu vaccines are developed in advance. Each year, WHO evaluates its influenza virus data, determines which three strains of seasonal flu will be prevalent in the coming flu season, and orders a vaccine that includes all three. Because pandemic flu strains result from antigenic shifts that cannot be anticipated, there is no possibility of predicting a pandemic strain and stockpiling doses in advance to ward off a pandemic. Public health experts can only respond to the emergence of a pandemic strain and begin developing a vaccine after it arrives. Thus it is crucial to have a vaccine development and production system primed and ready to begin at any moment.

In 2006 Congress authorized $3.3 billion for influenza pandemic preparedness. With these funds the government created incentives and grants to help the vaccine industry, and the U.S. Food and Drug Administration (FDA) streamlined the approval process for influenza vaccines, making vaccine research and development less costly. As a result of these policy changes, "the vaccine industry has undergone a renaissance in recent years,"[44] says Scott Gottlieb, a resident fellow at the American Enterprise Institute, a conservative public policy organization. As recently as 2004, he writes, most vaccines for U.S. consumers were made by 2 companies, only 1 of which was based in the United States. By 2009 there were 5 companies making H1N1 flu vaccines. Thus the nation's capacity to produce doses of vaccine against an influenza pandemic has significantly increased.

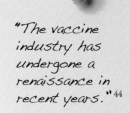

"The vaccine industry has undergone a renaissance in recent years." [44]

— Scott Gottlieb, resident fellow at the American Enterprise Institute, a conservative public policy organization.

A Lengthy Process

Even with more companies producing vaccines, serious challenges remain. The main issue is the time it takes to produce a vaccine. Vaccines are grown in live chicken eggs. First, the wild virus strain—that is, the virus as it occurs in nature—must be converted to a weaker strain that will not kill the chicken eggs. This strain, known as a seed strain, is then grown in the eggs, producing antigens that are needed to create an effective vaccine. It takes 5 to 7 weeks to develop the seed strain; it takes another 8 weeks to grow the virus. Quality control measures add 1 to 2 weeks to the process. All together, it takes 4 to 6 months to produce a vaccine. In most cases the first wave of a pandemic will have peaked during that time period, thus rendering vaccines an ineffective solution at least during the first wave of an influenza pandemic.

This is what happened during the H1N1 pandemic of 2009. Manufacturers started making vaccine in May; the first vaccines became available 5 months later, in October. At the end of the year (7 months after the start of production), 85 million doses had been developed, enough for only 28 percent of the U.S. population. By that time, the first wave of the pandemic had passed, although the pandemic level remained at phase 6 and

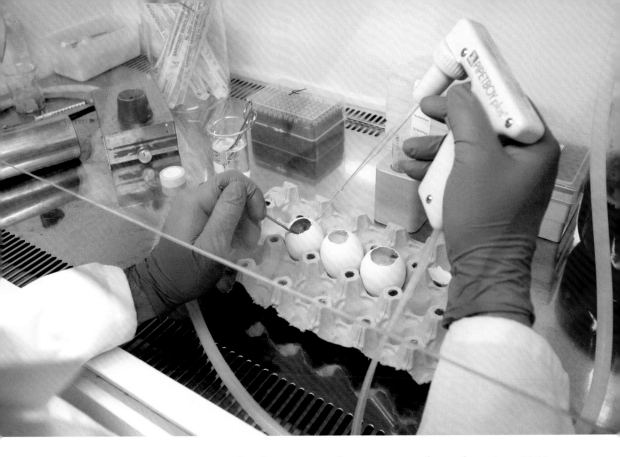

A technician cultures viruses in chicken eggs. This process takes many weeks, which lessens the likelihood of a new vaccine being developed in time for the first wave of an influenza pandemic. This is what happened in the case of the H1N1 vaccine.

H1N1 was the dominant influenza strain through spring 2010. Globally, availability of the H1N1 vaccine varied from region to region. WHO initiated an effort to secure donations of vaccines from governments, manufacturers, and foundations. By October 2009, the agency had secured promises of 200 million doses for 95 low and middle-income nations with a goal of immunizing 10 percent of their populations. By March 2010 WHO had delivered more than 10 million doses to 26 nations, including Afghanistan, Cambodia, and Nicaragua.

"Dirty, Slow and Expensive"

The use of chicken eggs to grow vaccines poses its own challenges. Millions of eggs are needed to produce enough doses to vaccinate the world. Dependence on these eggs is problematic. One risk is that the chickens producing the eggs could themselves be stricken by illness and die, reducing the number of eggs available for vaccine production. The chicken egg method is also expensive and lacking in flexibility. As Gottlieb puts it, "This chicken egg process is dirty, slow and expensive, costing more than $300 million to build a new plant and requiring more than five years to bring it online."[45]

The difficulty of the vaccine industry in responding to a pandemic is compounded by the fact that the same manufacturers who produce pandemic vaccines also produce seasonal flu vaccines. They cannot create adequate supplies of both seasonal flu vaccines and pandemic flu vaccines at the same time. Depending on the timing of a pandemic, officials sometimes have to decide between one or the other. As Gottlieb puts it, "A pandemic strain could emerge at the beginning of the production cycle for the seasonal vaccine. This would force a hard decision whether to shift some of the production capacity for a seasonal vaccine into efforts to manufacture a vaccine against pandemic viruses."[46] This decision would be a gamble, due to the unknowns surrounding pandemic viruses. Putting resources into creating a vaccine for a pandemic flu that proves mild could place many people at risk for seasonal flu who otherwise would have been vaccinated. Conversely, putting resources into the seasonal flu would leave people more vulnerable to a potentially deadly pandemic strain.

Improving the Vaccine Production Process

In response to these problems surrounding the vaccine production process, experts propose various solutions. One possibility is the use of adjuvants, additives that boost the power of the vaccine, allowing for smaller doses and stretching the supply to cover more people with less vaccine. Adjuvants, which could increase the strength of influenza vaccine by a factor of five, have been approved for use in Europe; however, the FDA has not approved adjuvants for use in the United States because the agency has not established their safety and efficacy.

Public health officials also call for alternative ways to grow vaccines. Some researchers are looking into the use of genetic engineering technologies, while others are exploring the possibility of growing the vaccine in animal cells instead of eggs. Cell-based production could cut 3 to 4 weeks from the process. This procedure is also faster to set up due to the lack of a need for millions of eggs.

What Is a Flu Vaccine?

A vaccine is a medicine that increases a person's immunity to a disease. In most cases it is made from a weakened form of the bug (either a virus or bacterium) that causes the disease itself. Once it enters the body, usually by means of injection, the vaccine stimulates the immune system, producing antibodies that attack and destroy the bug. If the body encounters the bug again in the future, its immune system again attacks and kills it. In this way the vaccine makes the vaccinated person more immune to the disease.

Every flu season, the World Health Organization identifies three strains of influenza that it believes pose the greatest threat to humans in the coming winter. Various drug companies around the world then produce a vaccine, known as a trivalent vaccine, against these three most likely candidates for the seasonal flu. If a new pandemic strain is discovered in time, it can be included in the seasonal vaccine; if not, a separate vaccine must be developed to fight it. Most influenza vaccine contains killed (or inactivated) virus and is delivered via an injection. However, it also comes in a live (or activated) form that is sprayed into the patient's nasal passage.

Tevi Troy, the former deputy director of the U.S. Department of Health and Human Services, describes some of the advantages of cell-based vaccine development over the egg-based process: "Eggs are . . . perishable, whereas cell lines can be frozen and maintained for a long time. Cell-based vaccines are also easier to create from a technical point of view, as growing virus strains in eggs makes the process longer and more complicated. Finally, people allergic to eggs can use the cell-based, but not the egg-based, vaccines."[47]

Several drug companies are already working on setting up cell-based vaccine manufacturing operations in the United States and elsewhere in the world. However, like adjuvants, they have not been approved by the FDA.

In addition to using adjuvants and cell-based technologies, many advocate the development of a universal vaccine that would be effective against all influenza strains—including pandemic strains. This vaccine would work by targeting the more stable parts of the flu virus rather than the parts that undergo major mutations. A universal vaccine would eliminate the need to create new seasonal vaccines each year. More important, it would allow officials to respond to a pandemic threat immediately rather than waiting the 4 to 6 months required by the current egg-based process. Experts believe that a universal vaccine is a realistic goal that could be achieved with major government investment. As stated by John M. Barry, the author of *The Great Influenza: The Story of the Deadliest Pandemic in History*, "Enough work has been done to suggest that this Holy Grail is achievable. Had influenza been taken seriously for the past 30 years, we would probably have [a universal vaccine] by now."[48]

Are Flu Vaccines Effective?

Even if new processes for developing vaccines more quickly and efficiently can be devised, will this really help prevent a pandemic? Some researchers say no. They believe that the ability of a flu vaccine to prevent a pandemic is overstated. Studies have shown that people who get a seasonal flu shot are half as likely to die during the following winter as people who do not get vaccinated. However, some skeptics have challenged the validity of these studies. They point out that many of the deaths of unvaccinated people were not caused by the flu or even complications from the flu; rather, they were caused by illnesses or injuries unrelated to flu.

Lisa Jackson, a physician and researcher with the Group Health Research Center in Seattle, found that vaccinations for seasonal flu may have no effect on mortality. Comparing the death rates of people who did and did not get flu shots, she found that those who got flu shots were less likely to die even before flu season. From her data, Jackson concludes that the flu vaccine appears to be effective because healthy people—who are more likely to survive with or without the vaccine—are more likely to get vaccinated. This phenomenon is known as the "healthy-user effect." Thus the statistics showing that people who do not get vaccinated are more likely to die may merely reflect the fact that people who decline vaccination are less healthy in general. According to Shannon Brownlee and Jeanne Lenzer, authors of an *Atlantic* magazine article on the topic, "The healthy-user effect explained the entire benefit that other researchers were attributing to flu vaccine, suggesting that the vaccine itself might not reduce mortality at all."[49]

> "The healthy-user effect explained the entire benefit that other researchers were attributing to flu vaccine, suggesting that the vaccine itself might not reduce mortality at all."[49]
>
> — Shannon Brownlee, senior research fellow at the New America Foundation, and Jeanne Lenzer, investigative journalist.

In Defense of Vaccine Effectiveness

The majority of researchers and public health experts believe that influenza vaccines are effective. The CDC states, "Influenza vaccination is the most effective method for preventing influenza and influenza-related complications."[50] WHO concurs: "Vaccination is the most effective way to prevent infection."[51]

Recent studies support the views of the CDC and WHO. A 2007 study published in the prestigious *New England Journal of Medicine* examined data from 10 flu seasons and found that vaccination was associated with a 27 percent reduction in the risk of hospitalization for pneumonia or influenza and a 48 percent reduction in the risk of death. In addition, a 2009 study published in *PLoS ONE*, a widely respected medical journal, found that influenza vaccines were effective in 53 percent of elderly Australian patients. In short, while the effectiveness of an influenza vaccine depends on many variables—including the ability to target the correct virus strain and the age and health of the person getting the vaccine—most agree it is the best way to keep people from getting sick and spreading the illness.

Debating the Safety of Vaccines

If having enough vaccine (and having it quickly) is one essential component of preparing for a pandemic, actually getting people to get vaccinated is another. Over the years, a small but vocal group of Americans has questioned the safety of vaccines, including those aimed at preventing influenza. Concerns about vaccine safety are fueled in part by events that occurred in 1976. During that year a new strain of H1N1 killed 1 soldier, prompting President Gerald Ford to call for the vaccination of the entire U.S. population to protect against what was thought to be a pandemic in the making. As it turned out, no pandemic actually occurred. Relief was short-lived, however, as it became known that approximately 500 of the 45 million Americans who had been vaccinated had apparently suffered serious side effects from the vaccine. They had developed Guillain-Barré syndrome (GBS), an autoimmune disorder that can cause paralysis and death. Although the number of people who actually contracted GBS was quite low—1 in 100,000—this episode left many people wary of the safety of vaccines.

Many studies have since investigated the link between the influenza vaccine and GBS. According to the CDC, most have found no connection, while two studies found that an extremely small number of patients—1 in 1 million—who receive the vaccine may have an increased risk of GBS. Other studies found a greater risk of getting GBS from influenza than from the influenza vaccine.

Questions About Thimerosal

At the center of concerns about vaccine safety is a preservative known as thimerosal, which kills bacteria and fungi. Thimerosal is composed of 49.6 percent mercury, a metal that is extremely hazardous to humans and can cause neurological problems or even death if ingested, inhaled, or absorbed through the skin in large enough amounts. Poisoning with mercury has been linked to cardiovascular disease, autism, seizures, mental retardation, and other neurological disorders. Some forms of the influenza vaccine contain no thimerosal, while others contain it at minute concentrations of 0.003 percent to 0.01 percent. Currently, the seasonal influenza vaccine contains thimerosal, although some seasonal vaccine doses contain only a trace of the substance and are considered thimerosal free. Some of the injectable doses of the H1N1 virus were thimerosal free, as were all of the nasal spray doses. The FDA and the CDC say that the level of mercury contained in all of these vaccines is harmless.

Pregnancy and the Influenza Vaccine

Pregnant women are among the groups considered at high risk for complications from influenza. They are vulnerable to secondary infections such as pneumonia because their immune system is suppressed in order to protect the fetus and because pregnancy makes it hard for them to clear their lungs. Aubrey Opdyke provides a vivid example of the harms that influenza can cause during pregnancy. After contracting the H1N1 virus in June 2009 (before a vaccine was available), the 27-year-old expectant mother was hospitalized for nearly 4 months, suffering a 5-week coma, collapsed lungs, and a seizure that nearly killed her. Her baby, delivered by cesarean section 10 to 14 weeks early, did not survive.

As tragic as Opdyke's story is, it could have been worse. As of August 2009 pregnant women accounted for 6 percent of deaths from H1N1, although pregnant women make up only 1 percent of the population. In an attempt to prevent such tragedies, the Centers for Disease Control and Prevention recommends that pregnant women get vaccinated for both seasonal and pandemic flu. However, only 15 percent of pregnant women choose to be vaccinated in any given year, compared with 30 percent of the general population.

As stated by the CDC's Advisory Committee on Immunization Practices, "No scientifically conclusive evidence exists of harm from exposure to thimerosal preservative–containing vaccine. . . . Therefore, the benefits of influenza vaccination outweigh the theoretical risk, if any, of thimerosal exposure through vaccination."[52]

Despite the lack of evidence that thimerosal contained in flu vaccines poses any risk to children or adults, a small percentage of the public is likely to resist any attempts at mass vaccination in the event of an influenza pandemic. In fact, those who oppose vaccines on the grounds of thimerosal risk are unlikely to be mollified by government assurances that vaccines are thimerosal free. In short, many people simply distrust the government enough to reject any vaccination effort. Polls illustrate this public skepticism regarding influenza pandemic vaccines. An October 2009 CBS News poll found that only 46 percent were likely to get the vaccine, and only 60 percent of parents were likely to get their children vaccinated. When asked why they would decline the vaccine, many people expressed doubts about its safety and effectiveness.

Should Vaccination Be Mandatory?

In the event of a deadly pandemic, one option would be for the government to require all citizens to be vaccinated. The U.S. Supreme Court opened the door for such a policy when it ruled in *Jacobsen v. Massachusetts* (1905) that the federal government could not prevent a state from requiring citizens to be vaccinated when the state deemed it necessary. However, it is unlikely that either the states or the federal government would take such a step.

The potential controversy over mandatory vaccination was demonstrated when New York attempted to require health-care workers to be vaccinated against the H1N1 virus during the 2009 pandemic. Because health-care workers come into contact with large numbers of people who are vulnerable to complications from the flu, public health experts contend that they should be among the first to be vaccinated against both seasonal and pandemic flu strains. If these workers are not vaccinated, there is a greater risk that they will contract the virus and spread it to their patients, who are at a higher risk of developing serious complications or even dying from the flu. In most years about 50 percent of health-care workers choose not to get vaccinated against the seasonal flu, although some voluntary programs have compliance rates as high as 80 percent.

In August 2009 New York State changed its laws to require most health-care workers to receive vaccinations against both seasonal flu and the H1N1 virus. Health-care organizations in Iowa and Washington proposed similar mandatory vaccination policies.

"Influenza vaccination is the most effective method for preventing influenza and influenza-related complications."[50]

— Centers for Disease Control and Prevention, the department of the U.S. government responsible for monitoring disease outbreaks and coordinating the government's response.

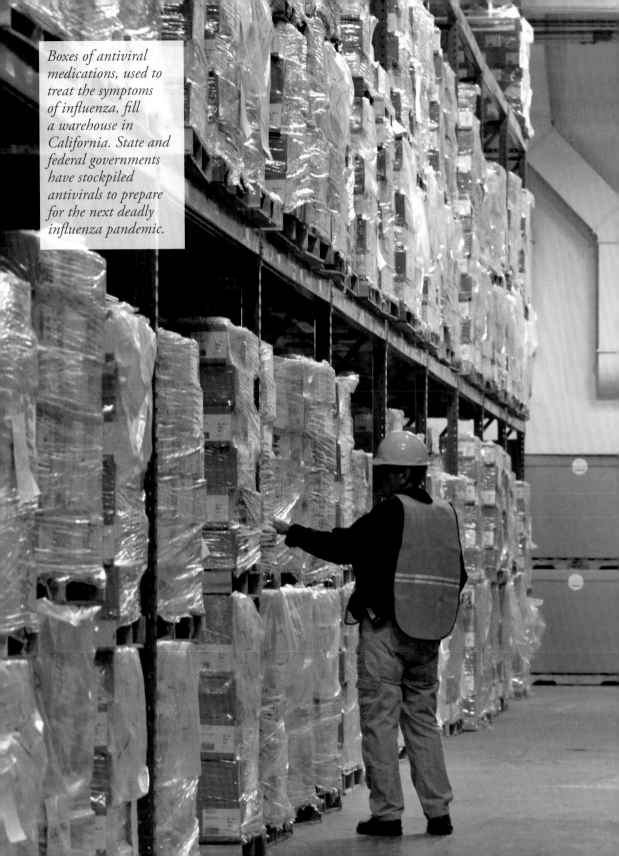

Boxes of antiviral medications, used to treat the symptoms of influenza, fill a warehouse in California. State and federal governments have stockpiled antivirals to prepare for the next deadly influenza pandemic.

These measures were promoted as a way to protect patients from infection by health-care workers and prevent the spread of disease and death. As stated by Christine J. Nutty, a registered nurse and the president of the Association for Professionals in Infection Control and Epidemiology, "Until vaccines are mandated for all health care providers, every patient will be placed at risk, many will develop influenza, and thousands will die."[53]

Opposition to Mandatory Vaccination

In New York many health-care workers opposed the new law. They staged protests and took the issue to court, arguing that the policy violated their right to make individual choices about their health care. In addition, because the law made no exception for people whose religious or cultural beliefs opposed immunization, workers with these beliefs would be forced out of their jobs. Thus the new policy could potentially deprive people of their livelihood and reduce the number of health-care workers available at a time when they are most needed. The New York Committee for Occupational Safety and Health, a coalition of unions and other organizations representing health-care workers in New York, argued that among other problems, the policy "removes an unknown number of the healthcare providers from the workforce. At a time when there will be a surge of patients with seasonal flu, and perhaps an additional surge because of the H1N1 virus, the loss of these healthcare providers will decrease the surge capability of affected facilities."[54]

In the face of mounting opposition, New York suspended the mandatory vaccination program. This episode illustrates the potential conflict that could result if the federal or state governments attempted to require large groups of citizens to be vaccinated against a pandemic flu strain.

Antiviral Drugs: The Second Line of Defense

In addition to vaccines, antiviral drugs are also used to fight the spread of influenza. While vaccines (the first line of defense) are given to healthy people to prevent them from getting the disease, antiviral drugs (the second line of defense) are given to those who already have the disease, in an attempt to shorten its duration, reduce the severity of symptoms, and prevent complications such as pneumonia. The 2 main antiviral drugs used for influenza are oseltamivir and zanamivir, which are more commonly known by their brand names, Tamiflu and Relenza. Both the CDC and WHO recommend giving antivirals to patients who are seriously ill and at risk for complications, preferably within the first 48 hours of illness. Doing so can shorten the length of illness by 1 to 2 days and reduce the chances the ill person will spread the virus to others, according to the CDC.

Following the avian influenza scare in the first decade of the twenty-first century, governments around the world stockpiled around 250 million courses of antiviral treatment (each patient must take multiple doses as part of treatment). By 2009 the U.S. government had 50 million courses of antivirals in its Strategic National Stockpile and had paid for an additional 22 million courses for state stockpiles. Experts believe that antivirals are an essential part of the pandemic flu defense, especially since vaccines would likely not be available in the first few months of an outbreak. As stated by John E. Calfee, a resident scholar at the American Enterprise Institute, "Antivirals can substantially and perhaps decisively reduce the scope and lethality of . . . outbreaks."[55]

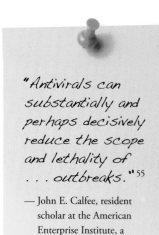

Government Preparation Versus Public Resistance

Due to vaccine development in recent years, humanity is at least partially prepared for a deadly pandemic. The world's capacity to produce vaccines has increased, although the process is still slow and vulnerable to disruption. Improved methods such as cell-based technologies and adjuvants could help speed up the process and increase the amount of vaccine available to the public. However, some segments of the public remain skeptical about the safety and effectiveness of influenza vaccines—especially if the vaccine is developed quickly and appears to be rushed through the safety testing process. Thus, if confronted by a deadly pandemic, governments may find that their efforts to control the spread of the virus and prevent widespread illness and death are hampered by public resistance.

Facts

- According to an October 2009 Rasmussen poll, 78 percent of Americans believe flu vaccines are at least somewhat effective at preventing flu outbreaks; 13 percent say they are not very effective or not at all effective.

- In a typical year only 30 percent of the population gets a flu vaccination, according to the Centers for Disease Control and Prevention.

- According to the Centers for Disease Control and Prevention, the effectiveness of the seasonal flu vaccine can range from as low as 30 percent to as high as 90 percent, depending on how well the vaccine matches the virus.

- In addition to easing influenza symptoms, antiviral drugs are also able to prevent a patient from developing the flu. According to the Centers for Disease Control and Prevention, antivirals can be from 70 percent to 90 percent effective against some strains of influenza.

- In a May 2009 Zogby poll, 36 percent of adults said they received an influenza vaccine for the current flu season.

How Effective Are Social Containment Measures?

In June 2009 members of a Southern California high school group became ill while in China on a school-sponsored trip. Under China's strict pandemic flu policy, they were quickly hospitalized and tested for the H1N1 virus. Five students and 1 teacher tested positive for the virus and were held in the hospital for treatment. The remaining members of their group were quarantined in a hotel. In all, 25 students and 4 teachers were each given a room with a telephone and television. They were forbidden to leave their rooms or to have physical contact with one another or anyone else. They could communicate only via telephone or by speaking through their open doorways. After 1 week free of flu symptoms, they were released and allowed to return to the United States.

The California students were not the only foreign travelers to be quarantined in China during the H1N1 pandemic. Many others from around the world—including New Orleans mayor C. Ray Nagin—experienced similar treatment. By the end of October, more than 2,000 Americans had been quarantined in China, with more than 200 testing positive for the H1N1 virus. The Chinese government insisted that its H1N1 quarantine measure was a necessary and effective way to protect the public from the spread of the disease. In June 2009 Mao Quan'an, a spokesperson for the

Chinese Health Ministry, stated, "We think that the method we are using has been pretty successful."[56]

What Is Social Containment?

China's quarantine of foreign travelers is just one example of a social containment measure. The phrase *social containment* is used to describe attempts to prevent the spread of a pandemic virus by means of limiting people's movements. It is thought that by isolating infected people and minimizing human-to-human contact, it may be possible to slow the spread of the virus from one geographical area to another or to reduce the

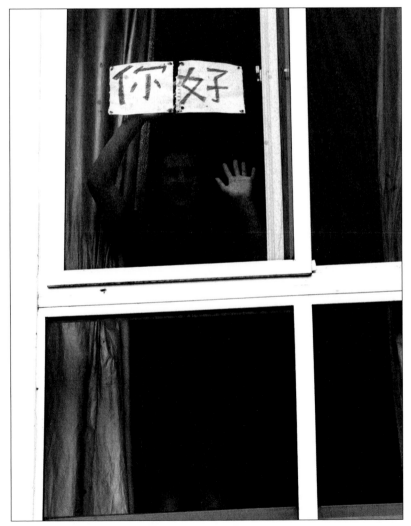

A student from the Southern California high school group that was quarantined in China in June 2009 holds up a sign that says hello *in Chinese. When some members of the group tested positive for the H1N1 virus, Chinese authorities quarantined all of them.*

Nonpharmaceutical Interventions to Slow the Spread of Flu

During the 2009 H1N1 pandemic flu outbreak, the U.S. government recommended the following behaviors to reduce the spread of disease:

- Cover your nose and mouth with a tissue when you cough or sneeze. Throw the tissue in the trash after you use it.

- Wash your hands often with soap and water, especially after you cough or sneeze. Alcohol-based hand cleaners are also effective.

- Avoid touching your eyes, nose, or mouth. Germs spread this way.

- Try to avoid close contact with sick people.

- Stay home if you are sick until at least 24 hours after you no longer have a fever (100°F or 37.8°C) or signs of a fever (without the use of a fever-reducing medicine, such as Tylenol).

- Follow public health advice regarding school closures, avoiding crowds and other social distancing measures.

- If you must have close contact with a sick person (for example, holding a sick infant), try to wear a facemask or N95 disposable respirator.

Centers for Disease Control and Prevention, "Prevention & Treatment," Flu.gov, January 8, 2010. www.pandemicflu.gov.

number of people infected within a community. In addition to quarantine, examples of social containment measures include closing schools, businesses, and public gathering places such as restaurants, churches, and movie theaters. Social containment falls within a broader category of flu-fighting strategies known as nonpharmaceutical interventions (NPIs). At the level of the individual, NPIs include frequent hand washing, covering one's face when coughing and sneezing, refraining from touching other people, and staying home when sick.

Can Pandemic Influenza Viruses Be Contained?

Some people believe that social containment measures can slow the spread of a virus as well as prevent an influenza pandemic. They posit that when a new virus emerges with the potential to create a pandemic, experts can move quickly to impose NPIs and keep people confined to a small area. In this way the outbreak may be limited to an epidemic, infecting people in one country or region, and will not cross borders and oceans to spread globally.

Preventing pandemics in this way would require constant surveillance of viruses around the world. Officials would have to pay special attention to the regions where new viruses typically emerge—undeveloped nations in which people live in close contact with animals. Some scientists contend that by closely monitoring these areas, new flu viruses can be spotted early, allowing for rapid deployment of virus control measures. Nathan Wolfe, a professor of epidemiology at the Johns Hopkins Bloomberg School of Public Health, has been studying virus outbreaks among hunters in Cameroon for 10 years. He contends, "By monitoring people who are exposed to animals in such viral hotspots, we can capture viruses at the very moment they enter human populations, and thus develop the ability to predict and perhaps even prevent pandemics."[57]

While all agree that it is important to conduct surveillance and to respond as quickly as possible to an outbreak, many are skeptical about the possibility of preventing a pandemic using such methods. One reason for their doubt is that pandemic flu strains are by definition highly transmissible and evasive, easily spreading quickly from person to person. Another reason for doubt is that influenza viruses do, in fact, emerge in remote, undeveloped regions that lack sophisticated public health facilities and communications networks. Henry I. Miller, a physician, molecular biologist, and fellow at Stanford University's Hoover Institution, explains why he believes preventing a pandemic at its source is not likely:

> Conditions in many countries are conducive to the emergence of . . . flu viruses, which mutate rapidly and inventively. Intensive animal husbandry procedures that place poultry and swine in close proximity to humans, combined with unsanitary conditions, poverty and grossly inadequate public-health infrastructure of all kinds . . . make it unlikely that a pandemic can be prevented or contained at the source.[58]

Can Quarantines Stop an Influenza Pandemic?

Quarantines are just one type of social containment measure. Quarantines, such as China's restriction of air travelers, are typically used not to prevent a pandemic but to slow the spread of a pandemic virus and limit the number of people stricken. However, in theory, once a virus has emerged and begun to spread, it is possible to stop it from entering a geographical area by means of quarantine. If no person carrying the virus is allowed into an area, there is no way for the virus to spread there. In his book *The Great Influenza: The Story of the Deadliest Pandemic in History*, John M. Barry describes how the Spanish flu virus of 1918 to 1920 spread from city to city in the United States. In rural Colorado, the towns located in the San Juan Mountains were remote enough that they had time to prepare for the disease. Although various towns, including Silverton and Ouray, instituted quarantines and closed businesses, the disease struck them one by one. However, the town of Gunnison was the exception, as Barry explains:

> Gunnison decided to isolate itself entirely. Gunnison lawmen blocked all through roads. Train conductors warned all passengers that if they stepped foot on the platform in Gunnison to stretch their legs, they would be arrested and quarantined for five days. Two Nebraskans trying simply to drive through to a town in the next county ran the blockade and were thrown into jail.[59]

As a result of these measures, according to Barry, "Gunnison escaped without a death."[60]

The example of Gunnison suggests that completely preventing the incursion of pandemic flu into an area is possible. However, it also makes clear how difficult it is. Gunnison was a remote, rural, early-twentieth-century community. Nevertheless, it took extreme measures to prevent people from entering. Such an undertaking would be virtually impossible in a major modern city. As Jonathan M. Metzl, a professor of psychiatry and women's studies at the University of Michigan, puts it, "Pandemics show little respect for national borders in a globalized world."[61]

A Persistent Disease

Most public health experts agree that it is not possible to stop a pandemic influenza strain completely by means of quarantine or other social containment measures, for several reasons. First, a person with the virus can carry it for two days—and is typically contagious for one day—without showing symptoms. Therefore, every person is a potential carrier and would need to be kept out of the protected area. Second, pandemic flu strains spread so easily from person to person that they are virtually impossible to contain. Third, people are extremely mobile in today's world; once it emerges, the virus will be carried to all corners of the planet within days by people traveling by air. As stated by Miller, "The rapid and constant movement of goods and people around the world makes early containment [of a pandemic flu virus] virtually impossible."[62]

The history of the 2009 H1N1 virus illustrates how difficult it is to contain an influenza virus. The outbreak began in Mexico in March 2009. However, it took several weeks for officials to recognize the emergence of a new influenza strain. Mexico enacted drastic measures, closing schools, businesses, churches, and other public meeting places in the nation's capital, all of which took a heavy toll on the economy. But these actions came too late and were too spotty to prevent a pandemic, and the virus quickly spread to all corners of the world.

> "Pandemics show little respect for national borders in a globalized world."[61]
>
> — Jonathan M. Metzl, professor of psychiatry and women's studies at the University of Michigan.

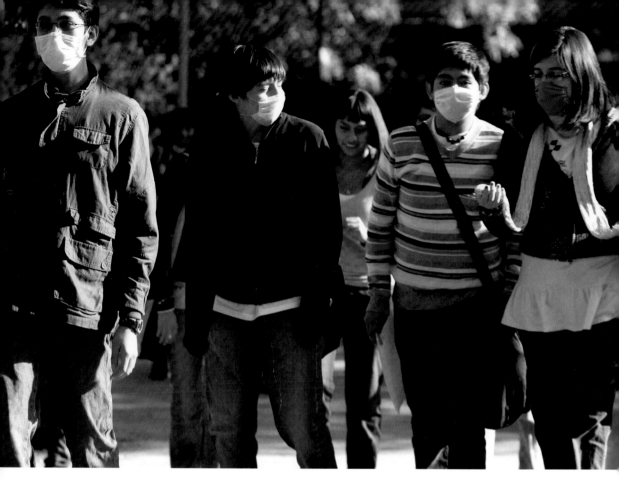

Students wearing masks as a precaution against H1N1 return to classes in Mexico City in May 2009. Mexican authorities closed schools, businesses, churches, and other public meeting places in an effort to halt the flu's spread.

Relying on air travel patterns from previous years, a group of Canadian researchers concluded that H1N1 had spread worldwide before public health officials even knew it existed. James Jay Carafano and Richard Weitz, writing in a paper published by the Heritage Foundation, a conservative think tank, stated that the H1N1 virus "had gone global before Mexican officials recognized that they had a serious problem. . . . Infected individuals likely crossed U.S. borders by land and air before H1N1 was identified."[63] Thus, imposing a quarantine would have done little to stop the H1N1 virus.

Social Containment to Reduce the Severity of a Pandemic

While quarantine and other social containment measures are unlikely to prevent a pandemic influenza virus from crossing national, state, and local borders, they can slow its progress so that fewer people become ill all at once. In this way they can lessen the burden the disease places on hospitals and public health systems. As Barry says, "The usefulness of non-pharmaceutical interventions is limited, and even if they work, their chief impact will be to flatten the pandemic's peak and stretch out the duration of a wave of illness to make it easier to handle."[64] For example, while China's quarantine measures did not keep the H1N1 virus out of the country in 2009, they may have saved lives. Because different countries use different techniques for identifying cases and deaths related to H1N1, making comparisons between countries is difficult. However, there is some indication that China may have been hit less hard by the virus than other nations. By November 2009 China had identified 59,000 cases of H1N1 and 30 deaths. By contrast, India had reported 500 deaths, and the United States had reported 2 million cases and 4,000 deaths. Thus social containment measures may have reduced the impact of the pandemic on the population.

Historical research supports the conclusion that social containment measures can reduce the impact of pandemic influenza. Two studies published in 2007 in the *Proceedings of the National Academies of Science* examined the use of measures such as closing schools, theaters, churches, and dance halls during the Spanish flu pandemic of 1918. Both studies found that U.S. cities that imposed measures early in the outbreak had fewer deaths than those that imposed such measures later in the outbreak. For example, Philadelphia waited more than 2 weeks after the first illness to impose social containment measures, whereas St. Louis imposed them within 2 days. Consequently, the peak weekly mortality rate (that is, the highest weekly number of deaths reported during the pandemic) was 8 times higher in Philadelphia than in St. Louis.

However, while peak mortality rates were dramatically different, overall mortality rates (that is, rates for the entire pandemic) were not significantly lower in cities that imposed social containment measures early. Once the measures were relaxed, rates of illness and death quickly rose in cities that had been relatively disease free. This result illustrates the tenacity of pandemic influenza. It also suggests that to be truly effective, social containment measures would need to be in place for a long time—perhaps as long as six months, the time it takes to develop a vaccine. Nevertheless, based on this research, some experts conclude that in the case of a truly deadly pandemic, imposing social containment measures early and sustaining them until a vaccine can be created could save many lives. As stated by Anthony S. Fauci, the director of the National Institutes of Health's National Institute of Allergy and Infectious Diseases: "A primary lesson of the 1918 influenza pandemic is that it is critical to intervene early. . . . Nonpharmaceutical interventions may buy valuable time at the beginning of a pandemic while a targeted vaccine is being produced."[65]

The Costs of Social Containment

Although social containment measures can slow the spread of a pandemic influenza virus, imposing significant constraints on people's ability to travel, work, and go to school—and maintaining such constraints for the needed length of time—is extremely difficult and costly. For example, it is estimated that the social containment measures Mexico imposed during the 2009 H1N1 outbreak cost the country billions of dollars. In addition, in 2003 China instituted similar measures in response to an outbreak of severe acute respiratory syndrome (SARS), a virus-caused disease that killed over 700 people. These measures cost the nation $50 billion, about 1 percent of its GDP. Hong Kong, whose economy is highly dependent on that of China's, lost 2.5 percent of its GDP.

In the United States it is estimated that the economic costs of social containment measures during a deadly flu pandemic would be significant. For example, researchers with the Brookings Institution, a public policy research organization that is generally considered politically centrist, calculated the cost to the nation of closing all schools in the country. Shutting down the schools would mean a loss of income for school employees as well as for parents forced to stay home to care for their children. The researchers found that closing all the schools for 4 weeks could cost between $10 billion and $47 billion. In addition, it would reduce key medical personnel by 6 percent to 19 percent (at a time when they are most in demand) due to the need for such workers to stay home with their children. If businesses such as restaurants, movie theaters, and sports venues were also closed, the economic impact would be staggering. In the case of a deadly pandemic, the challenge for governments would be to weigh the benefits in reduced illness and death that would result from social containment measures against the harms such a policy would impose on the economy and the disruptions it would cause to society in general.

Mexico City: Ghost Town

In the days after the emergence of the H1N1 virus in their country, Mexican officials imposed various social containment measures in Mexico City in an attempt to control the spread of the disease. CNN medical producer Danielle Dellorto, who rushed to the scene early in the outbreak, describes the city and the impact it had on her:

> Within 24 hours of arriving, the dense city of about 8 million people had figuratively turned into a ghost town. The mayor was urging people to stay inside; the hospitals were overcrowded; schools, public transportation, and restaurants closed their doors. At one point, I remember walking down the unusually empty streets of Mexico City in awe. It was an eerie feeling, but also a defining moment for me as a journalist. I realized that people, not just in Mexico City, were scared of this unknown killer virus. What was it? Would they be infected? What should they do? We didn't know it at the time, but H1N1 influenza was about to become a global epidemic and the world was already looking to us for answers.

Danielle Dellorto, "We Found Patient Zero; Here's How," Paging Dr. Gupta Blog, December 29, 2009. http://pagingdrgupta.blogs.cnn.com.

The Challenge of Imposing Social Containment Measures

In addition to burdening the economy, social containment measures would severely restrict people's freedom of movement, thereby affecting their quality of life. During the 2009 H1N1 outbreak, China was able to impose harsh restrictions in part because it has an authoritarian government and a citizenry used to complying with government directives—and perhaps fearful of disobeying such directives. Americans are accustomed to having the freedom to choose where and when to travel, whether to go to work or school, and what public places to frequent. Whether they would cooperate with government attempts to control their movements and contacts, especially if doing so would impact their lifestyle or livelihood for a long period of time, is open for debate. Americans, with their tradition of self-reliance, mistrust of authority, and independent spirit, seem unlikely to succumb to either fear of infection or fear of government warnings and threats.

Little was asked of Americans during the 2009 H1N1 pandemic. On April 26, 2009, the U.S. Department of Health and Human Services declared a public health emergency. This step gave the federal government the authority to impose quarantines, restrict the movement of people across borders, and shut down some public transportation systems. Because the virus appeared to be relatively mild, and because it had already spread quickly throughout the states, the government refrained from closing borders or restricting travel, although officials did isolate some immigrants and travelers who were believed to be infected with the virus. The CDC issued guidelines to the public on ways to avoid spreading the flu, such as frequent hand washing, covering one's coughs and sneezes, and staying home when ill. The CDC gave some inconsistent guidance on the issue of school closures in the early days of the pandemic. As a result, the policy on the closing of schools varied in different states, cities, and school districts. During the initial wave of the pandemic in the spring, many schools were closed for a significant amount of time. However, by the fall the CDC had clarified its

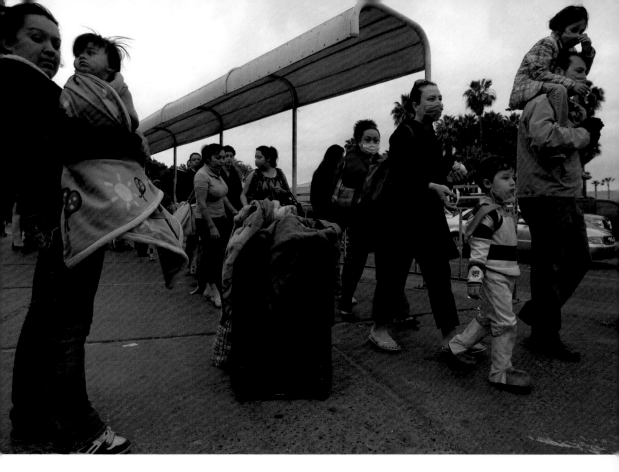

school closure recommendations, resulting in very few closures, and most businesses and public meeting places remained open throughout the pandemic. Thus, compared with the citizens of Mexico, Americans faced very few inconveniences during the H1N1 pandemic of 2009.

Ignoring Advice

Despite the lack of restrictions or impositions, many Americans accused the government of overreacting to the 2009 H1N1 pandemic. In addition, many people ignored even the seemingly reasonable advice to protect themselves from infection. It was reported that some people even tried to contract the virus by means of "swine flu parties," believing that if they became ill with the relatively mild H1N1strain they would be immune from a possibly more severe strain in the future (although the CDC strongly advised against having such "parties"). In addition, many Americans

Health officials believe that people crossing the U.S.-Mexico border probably helped to spread the H1N1 virus. Here, people pass through the Tijuana– San Diego border crossing, some wearing masks.

who were ill continued to go about their business even though they had been instructed to stay home. According to the Trust for America's Health, a nonprofit organization that advocates policies to protect public health, "There were numerous media reports of people with influenza-like illness continuing to go to work because they had no sick leave and feared losing their jobs, and some parents sent sick children to school because they could not say home to care for them."[66]

Based on the public's response to H1N1, according to the Trust for America's Health, "It became clear to officials how difficult it would be to carry out plans to limit mass gatherings or cancel major events if that became necessary."[67] Indeed, Americans' resistance to even the minor control measures instituted during the 2009 H1N1 virus suggests that in the case of a truly deadly pandemic, the necessary imposition of quarantines, closing of borders and businesses, and banning of mass public gatherings would face stiff opposition.

Preparing for the Worst

The insidious nature of the influenza virus makes it impossible to control completely. In fact, new strains emerge due precisely to the virus's evolutionary urge to survive and evade the body's immune responses. However, while social control measures are unlikely to stop the geological reach of a pandemic influenza virus completely, they can lessen the number of people infected at any one time and thereby allow public health experts to mount a more effective response. In the event of an extremely virulent strain of pandemic influenza, governments must be prepared to restrict travel between countries and reduce mass gatherings within their own borders by closing schools, restaurants, entertainment venues, workplaces, and other sites where people come in close contact. In addition, they must be ready to communicate effectively in order to convince the public that such controls imposed on their movements are genuinely warranted. These efforts could prevent suffering and prevent the loss of life in a deadly influenza pandemic.

"It became clear to officials [during the 2009 H1N1 pandemic] how difficult it would be to carry out plans to limit mass gatherings or cancel major events if that became necessary."[67]

— The Trust for America's Health, a nonprofit organization that advocates policies to protect public health.

Facts

- In a May 2009 Zogby poll, 40 percent of Americans said they were confident in the government's ability to handle a potential pandemic flu crisis; 35 percent said they were not confident.

- In a Rasmussen poll conducted on May 4, 2009, early in the H1N1 outbreak, 63 percent of Americans said the border with Mexico should be closed until the epidemic was under control.

- According to researchers at St. Michael's College in Canada, the five countries that received the most H1N1-infected air travelers from Mexico were the United States, Canada, France, Spain, and Germany.

- Mexico's finance minister estimates that social containment measures in response to the 2009 H1N1 pandemic cost the nation $2.3 billion, which represents 0.3 percent of the nation's gross domestic product.

- Fifty-eight percent of Americans say they would be willing to go into voluntary quarantine if asked, according to a May 2009 Zogby poll.

Related Organizations and Web Sites

American Public Health Association (APHA)
800 I St. NW
Washington, DC 20001
phone: (202) 777-2742
fax: (202) 777-2534
e-mail: comments@apha.org
Web site: www.apha.org

The APHA is an organization of public health professionals that aims to protect all Americans from preventable, serious health threats. It advocates community-based health promotion, disease prevention activities, and preventive health services, including vaccination as a means of preventing the spread of influenza.

American Red Cross
2025 E St. NW
Washington, DC 20006
phone: (202) 303-5000
Web site: www.redcross.org

The Red Cross is a nonprofit emergency response organization. It offers humanitarian care to the victims of war and natural disasters, including influenza pandemics. Its Web site offers fact sheets and guidelines on preparing for an influenza pandemic.

Centers for Disease Control and Prevention (CDC)
1600 Clifton Rd.
Atlanta, GA 30333

phone: (800) 232-4636
e-mail: cdcinfo@cdc.gov
Web site: www.cdc.gov

The CDC, part of the U.S. Department of Health and Human Services, is responsible for developing disease prevention and control measures to improve the health of Americans. It monitors influenza outbreaks and reports on rates of illness and death from the flu in the United States.

Flu.gov
Web site: www.pandemicflu.gov

Flu.gov is a Web site created by the U.S. Department of Health and Human Services to provide information on seasonal, H1N1 (swine), H5N1 (bird), and pandemic influenza for the general public, health and emergency preparedness professionals, policy makers, government and business leaders, school systems, and local communities.

National Institutes of Health (NIH)
9000 Rockville Pike
Bethesda, MD 20892
phone: (301) 496-4000
e-mail: nihinfo@od.nih.gov
Web site: www.nih.gov

The NIH, a part of the U.S. Department of Health and Human Services, is the primary federal agency for conducting and supporting medical research. The NIH oversees research into the effectiveness of vaccines and antiviral drugs to prevent and treat influenza. Its Web site offers information on influenza.

National Vaccine Information Center (NVIC)
407-H Church St.
Vienna, VA 22180
phone: (703) 938-0342
fax: (703) 938-5768
e-mail: contactnvic@gmail.com
Web site: www.nvic.org

The NVIC is a nonprofit organization that advocates vaccine safety and informed consent in the vaccination system. It neither promotes the use of vaccines nor advises against their use. It supports the availability of all preventive health-care options, including vaccination, and the right of consumers to make educated, voluntary health-care choices.

Prevent Childhood Influenza

Childhood Influenza Immunization Coalition
139 Fifth Ave., 3rd floor
New York, NY 10010
phone: (212) 886-2277
e-mail: ciic@nfid.org
Web site: www.preventchildhoodinfluenza.org

Prevent Childhood Influenza is a group of more than 30 American public health, medical, patient, and parent groups that are committed to protecting children's health. As the Childhood Influenza Immunization Coalition, they seek to increase influenza immunization rates among children by promoting vaccination.

ThinkTwice Global Vaccine Institute

PO Box 9638
Santa Fe, NM 87504
e-mail: global@thinktwice.com
Web site: www.thinktwice.com

The ThinkTwice Global Vaccine Institute provides parents and other concerned people with educational resources, enabling them to make more informed vaccine decisions. It encourages an uncensored exchange of vaccine information and supports every family's right to accept or reject vaccines.

Trust for America's Health (TFAH)

1730 M St. NW, Suite 900
Washington, DC 20036
phone: (202) 223-9870
fax: (202) 223-9871
e-mail: info@tfah.org
Web site: www.healthyamericans.org

The TFAH is a nonprofit organization dedicated to improving the health of Americans and working to make disease prevention a national priority. Its Web site offers several reports on the H1N1 influenza pandemic and on U.S. influenza pandemic preparedness.

U.S. Department of Health and Human Services

200 Independence Ave. SW
Washington, DC 20201
phone: (877) 696-6775
Web site: www.hhs.gov

The U.S. Department of Health and Human Services is the U.S. government's principal agency for protecting the health of all Americans and providing essential human services. Its Web site offers guidance to health-care professionals and others on antiflu activities, including recommendations regarding vaccines and antiviral drugs.

World Health Organization (WHO)

Avenue Appia 20
1211 Geneva 27
Switzerland
phone: 41 22 791 21 11
fax: 41 22 791 31 11
e-mail: mediainquiries@who.int
Web site: www.who.int

WHO is the authority for health within the United Nations. It is responsible for providing leadership on global health matters, including influenza surveillance and education regarding emerging threats and pandemics. WHO's Web site offers a great deal of information for both professionals and laypersons.

Additional Reading

Books

Mark Honigsbaum, *Living with Enza: The Forgotten Story of Britain and the Great Flu Pandemic of 1918.* London: Macmillan, 2009.

Jeffrey R. Ryan, *Pandemic Influenza: Emergency Planning and Community Preparedness.* Boca Raton, FL: CRC, 2009.

Geary W. Sikich, *Protecting Your Business in a Pandemic: Plans, Tools, and Advice for Maintaining Business Continuity.* Westport, CT: Praeger, 2008.

Alan Sipress, *The Fatal Strain: On the Trail of Avian Flu and the Coming Pandemic.* New York: Viking, 2009.

David Waltner-Toews, *The Chickens Fight Back: Pandemic Panics and Deadly Diseases That Jump from Animals to Humans.* Vancouver, BC: Greystone, 2007.

Periodicals

Philip Alcabes, "5 Myths About Pandemic Panic," *Washington Post*, March 15, 2009.

Anne Applebaum, "A Panic to Welcome," *Washington Post*, May 12, 2009.

John M. Barry, "Invest in Vaccines to Avert Pandemic," *Atlanta Journal-Constitution*, July 1, 2009.

Shannon Brownlee and Jeanne Lenzer, "Does the Vaccine Matter?" *Atlantic*, November 2009.

Steve Chapman, "Overreacting to Swine Flu," *Reason*, May 4, 2009.

Michael Fumento, "Swine Flu Piglet 'Pandemic,'" *Washington Times*, October 20, 2009.

Henry I. Miller, "Understanding Swine Flu," *Wall Street Journal*, April 28, 2009.

Paul A. Offit, "Thimerosal and Vaccines—a Cautionary Tale," *New England Journal of Medicine*, September 27, 2007.

Michael T. Osterholm, "Unprepared for a Pandemic," *Foreign Affairs*, March/April 2007.

Michael Specter, "The Fear Factor," *New Yorker*, October 12, 2009.

Jennifer Steinhauer, "Swine Flu Shots Revive a Debate About Vaccines," *New York Times*, October 26, 2009.

Nathan Wolfe, "How to Prevent a Pandemic," *New York Times*, April 30, 2009.

Source Notes

Introduction: Preparing for the Inevitable

1. Margaret Chan, "World Now at the Start of 2009 Influenza Pandemic," World Health Organization, June 11, 2009. www.who.int.

2. President's Council of Advisors on Science and Technology, "Report to the President on U.S. Preparations for 2009-H1N1 Influenza," White House, August 7, 2009. www.whitehouse.gov.

3. Michael T. Osterholm, "Unprepared for a Pandemic," *Foreign Affairs*, March/April 2007, p. 47.

4. Osterholm, "Unprepared for a Pandemic," p. 47.

Chapter One: What Is the History of Influenza Pandemics?

5. President's Council of Advisors on Science and Technology, "Report to the President on U.S. Preparations for 2009-H1N1 Influenza."

6. Debbie Crane, "Edna Breedlove Clampitt," Pandemic Influenza Storybook. www.flu.gov.

7. World Health Organization, "Avian Influenza: Assessing the Pandemic Threat," January 2005. www.who.int.

8. Mark Honigsbaum, *Living with Enza: The Forgotten Story of Britain and the Great Flu Pandemic of 1918*. London: Macmillan, 2009, p. 15.

9. Honigsbaum, *Living with Enza*, p. 16.

10. Laurie Garrett, "The Next Pandemic?" *Foreign Affairs*, July/August 2005, p. 3.

11. Michael Specter, "The Fear Factor," *New Yorker*, October 12, 2009. www.newyorker.com.

12. Arthur Allen, "Figuring Out the Flu," *Los Angeles Times*, May 11, 2009, p. A23.

Chapter Two: Can Predictions Help the World Prepare for Future Pandemics?

13. World Health Organization, "Avian Influenza."

14. World Health Organization, "Avian Influenza."

15. Congressional Budget Office, "A Potential Influenza Pandemic: An Update on Possible Macroeconomic Effects and Policy Issues," July 27, 2006. www.cbo.gov.

16. American Federation of Labor and Congress of Industrial Organizations, "Healthcare Workers in Peril: Preparing to Protect Worker Health and Safety During Pandemic Influenza: A Union Survey Report," April 16, 2009. www.aflcio.org.

17. Homeland Security Council, "National Strategy for Pandemic Influenza," Flu.gov, November 2005. www.flu.gov.

18. Geary W. Sikich, *Protecting Your Business in a Pandemic: Plans, Tools, and Advice for Maintaining Business Continuity*. Westport, CT: Praeger, 2008, p. 175.

19. Warwick J. McKibbin and Alexandra A. Sidorenko, "The Global Costs of an Influenza Pandemic," *Milken Institute Review*, Third Quarter, 2007, p. 23.

20. McKibbin and Sidorenko, "The Global Costs of an Influenza Pandemic," p. 27.

21. Congressional Budget Office, "A Potential Influenza Pandemic."

22. Sikich, *Protecting Your Business in a Pandemic*, p. 174.

23. Sikich, *Protecting Your Business in a Pandemic*, p. 196.

24. U.S. House of Representatives Committee on Homeland Security, "Getting Beyond Getting Ready for Pandemic Influenza," January 2009. http://homeland.house.gov.

25. Sikich, *Protecting Your Business in a Pandemic*, p. 201.

26. Michael Fumento, "Swine Flu Piglet 'Pandemic,'" *Washington Times*, October 20, 2009, p. A-21.

27. *Christian Science Monitor*, "Swine Flu: A Plan, Not a Prediction," August 28, 2009, p. 8.

28. Anne Applebaum, "A Panic to Welcome," *Washington Post*, May 12, 2009. www.washingtonpost.com.

29. Garrett, "The Next Pandemic?" p. 3.

30. World Health Organization, "Avian Influenza."

31. Osterholm, "Unprepared for a Pandemic," p. 47.

Chapter Three: Is The Global Pandemic Response System Adequate?

32. Anne Applebaum, "Keep the Disease Fighters Focused," *Washington Post*, April 28, 2009. www.washingtonpost.com.

33. Lawrence Gostin, "Fighting the Flu with One Hand Tied," *Washington Post*, May 1, 2009, p. A-21.

34. Trust for America's Health, "Pandemic Flu Preparedness: Lessons from the Frontlines," issue brief, June 2009. http://healthy americans.org.

35. Vincent Racaniello , "WHO Will Redefine Pandemic," Virology Blog, May 23, 2009. www.virology.ws.

36. Gostin, "Fighting the Flu with One Hand Tied," p. A-21.

37. Richard Holbrooke and Laurie Garrett, "'Sovereignty' That Risks Global Health," *Washington Post*, August 10, 2008, p. B-7.

38. U.S. Department of Health and Human Services, *Pandemic Influenza Implementation Plan: Parts I and II*, November 2006. www.hhs.gov.

39. Trust for America's Health, "Pandemic Flu Preparedness."

40. President's Council of Advisors on Science and Technology, "Report to the President on U.S. Preparations for 2009-H1N1 Influenza."

41. U.S. House of Representatives Committee on Homeland Security, "Getting Beyond Getting Ready for Pandemic Influenza."

42. Nicole Lurie, "Safeguarding Our Nation: HHS Response to the H1N1 Outbreak," U.S. Department of Health and Human Services, October 27, 2009. www.hhs.gov.

43. Kim Krisberg, "Global Public Health Mobilizes to Confront H1N1 Flu Outbreak: Disease Brings Preparedness to the Forefront," *Nation's Health*, 2009. www.medscape.com.

Chapter Four: Can Vaccines Prevent a Pandemic?

44. Scott Gottlieb, "Vaccine Readiness in a Time of Pandemic: Policy Promises Realized and the Challenges That Remain," American Enterprise Institute for Public Policy Research, May 2009. www.aei.org.

45. Gottlieb, "Vaccine Readiness in a Time of Pandemic."

46. Gottlieb, "Vaccine Readiness in a Time of Pandemic."

47. Tevi Troy, "Developing a Better Vaccine," *Forbes*, September 27, 2009. www.forbes.com.

48. John M. Barry, "Invest in Vaccines to Avert Pandemic," *Atlanta Journal-Constitution*, July 1, 2009, p. A17.

49. Shannon Brownlee and Jeanne Lenzer, "Does the Vaccine Matter?" *Atlantic*, November 2009. www.theatlantic.com.

50. Centers for Disease Control and Prevention, National Center for Immunization and Respiratory Diseases, "Use of Influenza A (H1N1) 2009 Monovalent Vaccine: Recommendations of the Advisory Committee on Immunization Practices (ACIP), 2009," *Morbidity and Mortality Weekly Report*, August 28, 2009. www.cdc.gov.

51. World Health Organization, "Fact Sheet Number 211: Influenza (Seasonal)," April 2009. www.who.int.

52. Quoted in U.S. Food and Drug Administration, "Thimerosal in Vaccines: Questions and Answers," July 10, 2009. www.fda.gov.

53. Christine J. Nutty, "Should Health Care Workers Be Required to Be Immunized Against Influenza?" *Family Practice News*, October 1, 2009, p. 10.

54. New York Committee for Occupational Safety and Health, letter to Richard F. Daines, commissioner of the New York State Department of Health, New York State Nurse's Association, October 2, 2009. www.nysna.org.

55. John E. Calfee, "And Now, a Few Words About Antivirals for Pandemic Flu," American Enterprise Institute for Public Policy Research, June 2, 2009. www.aei.org.

Chapter Five: How Effective Are Social Containment Measures?

56. Quoted in Lucy Hornby, "China Credits Quarantine for Containing H1N1," Reuters, June 11, 2009. www.reuters.com.

57. Nathan Wolfe, "How to Prevent a Pandemic," *New York Times*, April 30, 2009, p. A-27.

58. Henry I. Miller, "Understanding Swine Flu," *Wall Street Journal*, April 28, 2009. http://online.wsj.com.

59. John M. Barry, *The Great Influenza: The Story of the Deadliest Pandemic in History*. New York: Penguin, 2005, p. 345.

60. Barry, *The Great Influenza*, p. 346.

61. Jonathan M. Metzl, "China's Flu Phobia," *Los Angeles Times*, July 12, 2009, p. A-24.

62. Miller, "Understanding Swine Flu."

63. James Jay Carafano and Richard Weitz, "Swine Flu: What Every American Should Know," Heritage Foundation, September 10, 2009. www.heritage.org.

64. Barry, "Invest in Vaccines to Avert Pandemic," p. A17.

65. Quoted in U.S. Department of Health and Human Services, "Rapid Response Was Crucial to Containing the 1918 Flu Pandemic," National Institutes of Health News, April 2, 2007. www3.niaid.nih.gov.

66. Trust for America's Health, "Pandemic Flu Preparedness."

67. Trust for America's Health, "Pandemic Flu Preparedness."

Index

and Technology (PCAST), 8, 11, 36, 37, 50–51
Proceedings of the National Academies of Science (journal), 75

quarantines
    effectiveness of, 72–73
    voluntary, willingness of Americans to go into during pandemic, 81
    See also social containment measures

Racaniello, Vincent, 44
Rasmussen Reports, 39, 67, 81
Relenza, 66
response planning, 50–51
    confidence in government for, 81
    importance of assumptions/predictions in, 26–27
    spending on, 21
    using scenarios for, 32

severe acute respiratory syndrome (SARS), 39, 45
Sidorenko, Alexandra A., 29, 33
Sikich, Geary W., 31, 34, 36
social containment measures, 69–71
    economic costs of imposing, 76–77
    in H1N1 pandemic in U.S., 78–79
    severity of pandemic and, 74–76
    See also quarantines
Spanish flu pandemic (1918–1920), 6–7, 11, 15–16
    isolation of virus causing, 15
    lessons of, 76
    response to, 17–18
Specter, Michael, 20
St. Michael's College (Canada), 81
Supari, Siti Fadilah, 45
surveillance. *See* influenza surveillance
surveys
    on Americans' concern for H1N1 outbreak, 53
    on confidence in government's ability to handle pandemic, 81
    of effectiveness of flu vaccines, 67
    on media exaggeration of H1N1 threat, 39
    on public resistance to H1N1 vaccination, 63

on willingness of Americans to go into voluntary quarantine during pandemic flu, 81
swine flu. *See* H1N1 (swine) influenza
swine flu scare (1976), 19–20, 60–61

Tamiflu, 66
thimerosal, 61–63
transmission rates, 13
Trust for America's Health, 50, 80

United States
    economic costs of social containment measures in, 76–77
    influenza surveillance in, 47–50
    number of H1N1 cases/deaths in, 75
    readiness for influenza pandemic in, 47–50
U.S. House of Representatives Committee on Homeland Security, 34–35, 51

vaccines/vaccination
    debate on safety of, 60–61
    effectiveness of, 59–60
    fear of, 20
    mandatory, opposition to, 65
    pregnancy and, 62
    production of, 55–56
        improving, 57–59
    risks of using chicken eggs to grow virus for, 56–57
    seasonal, percent of population receiving, 67

Weitz, Richard, 74
Wolfe, Nathan, 71
World Health Organization (WHO), 6, 8, 53
    Asian flu pandemic and, 19
    H1N1 flu pandemic and, 23, 43
    importance of, 40–42
    on influenza virus mutations and pandemics, 13
    phase system of, 42–44
    on scenarios for influenza preparedness, 32
    on unpredictability of influenza pandemics, 26

Zogby poll, 67, 81
    See also surveys

About the Author

Scott Barbour received a bachelor's degree in English and a master's degree in social work from San Diego State University. He has written and edited numerous books on social, historical, and mental health topics.